EAT GOOD OR DIE BAD

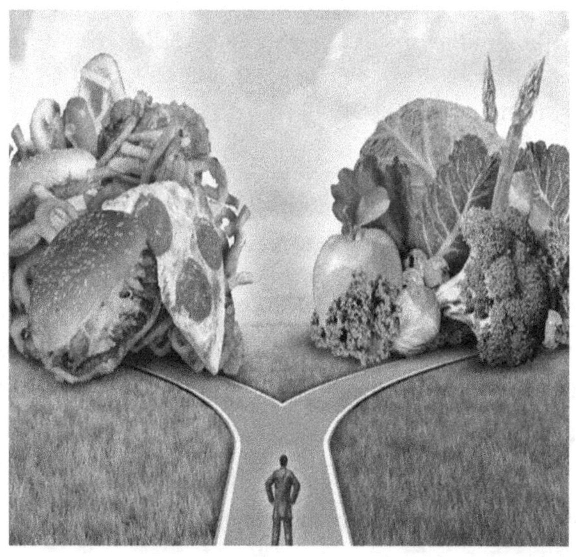

Scientifically Proven Diet for Balance, Optimum Health & Change your Eating Habits to Discover Lifelong Fitness

DR. ZAINAB ZAMAN

damages, or monetary loss due to the information herein, either directly or indirectly.

Respective authors own all copyrights not held by the publisher.

The information herein is offered for informational purposes solely, and is universal as so. The presentation of the information is without contract or any type of guarantee assurance.

The trademarks that are used are without any consent, and the publication of the trademark is without permission or backing by the trademark owner. All trademarks and brands within this book are for clarifying purposes only and are the owned by the owners themselves, not affiliated with this document.

YOUR FREE GIFT

I'd like to give you a free gift before we get started. It's my way of saying thank you for taking the time to read this book with me.

Your present is an exceptional food journal. This journal will:

- Allow you to keep track of calories and macronutrients (protein, fat, carbs, etc.) on a daily basis, as well as record meals and drinks.

- Make you accountable

- Help you understand where your calories are coming from

- Identify if any extra calories are sneaking back into your diet

- Act as a deterrent - just by knowing that you have to write it down suddenly makes that second helping not so important

- Provide you with a concrete record of your success

You typically set a daily calorie goal and use the food diary to help you meet that goal.

How can you obtain a copy of the food journal? It's simple. Visit my website (https://nutritionreads.com/) and sign-up for my mail list (or simply click on the link above). You will have direct access to the food journal in PDF format, which you can print at any time. It's all up to you.

You'll also be the first to know when I publish a new productive book if you join my email list. I plan to release them at a steep discount (or even free) for the first 24hours. You will receive an early notification if you sign up. It's perfectly good if you don't want to join my mailing list. It simply means that I need to win your trust. With that in mind, I believe you'll appreciate the information I've given in this food journal. I believe you will appreciate what I can offer you in your life.

Let's get started without further hesitation.

https://nutritionreads.com/free-gift/

Table of Contents

Introduction

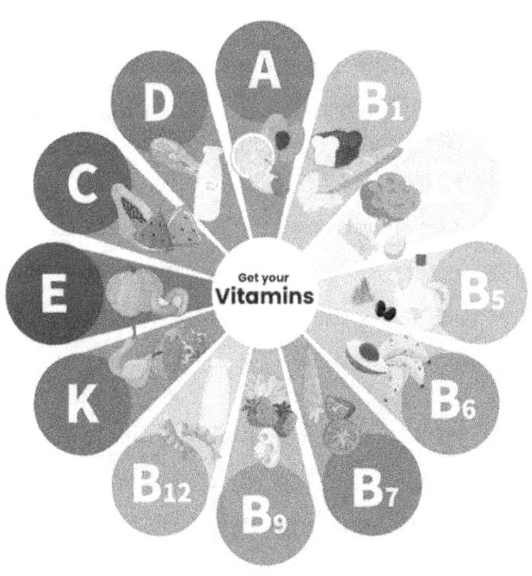

Developing and maintaining healthy eating habits is a way for you and your family to enhance your health, lifestyle, and appearance. It's amazing how once you make a habit of something, it is no longer difficult to keep doing it, and that goes for bad and good habits. Experts have shown that eating the right foods and exercising might be the secret to living a long, enjoyable, and successful life.

The human body is always inclined towards living a life that is both comfortable and healthy. We all want to feel soothed with certain comforts of our lives and like being surrounded by the best facilities in life. And this is when we say, "Health is Wealth." We can never enjoy anything in our lives if we are not physically or mentally healthy. This is why dieticians and doctors focus the most on a diet and whatever we consume throughout the day. If you are also facing your life issues and don't feel fit, you may need a revamp of your food intake.

We all ask ourselves about our health and why we face issues in certain parts of our lives. The answers to these questions are somehow influenced by what we eat and how we live our days.

Often our health needs more attention than regular days, and we get sensitive to external factors. In this period, our bodies can only fight off hypersensitivities with the energy of the right food and exercise that you may have done during regular days. As we enter into years of youth, we are always full of energy, and our body systems don't need much external aid to function well. But with the increasing years on the calendar of our lives, our internal health starts declining. We start feeling tired after a little workout, and we also think exhausted after waking up, even when we have a full sleep. This is why we begin needing changes in our diet so that our body systems can function correctly.

Our diet can do wonders for our bodies and the quality of life—no wonder human needs always fall back to good food and sound sleep. Often, we need a good diet so that our body can build up immunity levels and fight off against chronic illnesses. Our bodies can always fight against many illnesses when we have certain food items added to our diet to boost our immunity. You will get to know about certain chronic illnesses that can be fought well by having the proper diet in our food. We need to consume certain foods to build our energy against chronic illnesses and help us live a high-quality life.

This book is meant to be a road map of what to eat, focus on the best and current science. The most important thing you do every day is what you put on your fork. It affects your ability to live a rich, energetic, connected, soulful life, a life in which you have the energy to care about yourself, enjoy your friends and family, support your neighbor, turn up absolutely in the world for your work, and live your dreams. You are positively shaping all about you if you enjoy real, whole, nutritious meals that you prepare using real ingredients. To put it plainly, food is the key to living well and caring well, and solving all of what's wrong in our world.

Part 1

AN OVERVIEW OF ALL ESSENTIAL NUTRIENTS & VITAMINS

As you have always hazard 'You are what you eat!'. We are here with a detailed guide of what, when, and how you should have the nutrition your body needs.

Following are the 6 such nutrients and vitamins that your body needs frequently.

1. Carbohydrates: Carbs are essential for our bodies to help in the immune system's functioning, brain function, nervous system, and digestive system. The need is to limit simple carbs intake and start having complex carbs to help the bodily functions work better.

2. Protein: Protein is the micronutrient that each of our body cells needs to perform correctly. They help ensure the proper development and growth of bones, muscles, and hair. They also help form hormones, antibodies, and other essential substances.

3. Fats: You may think high-fat foods are harmful, but they are not. Our body needs a good supply of fats as well to work correctly. Fats help in cell growth, blood clotting, and the reduction of type 2 diabetes and heart illnesses.

4. Dietary Fiber: Using dietary supplements is ideal for obtaining the benefits of food items that you wouldn't otherwise get from the regular diet. It is suggested first to talk with your doctor before you start taking the supplements.

5. Vitamins: These are the micronutrients that our body needs to perform various bodily actions, including strengthening teeth and bones. Maintaining healthy skin, supporting healthy blood, etc.

6. Minerals: Minerals are another type of micronutrient that is the primary and trace minerals. The body needs to balance both of them, which helps the body balance its water levels, maintain a healthy skin tone, nails, and hair and improve bone health.

Explanation:

Carbohydrates:

What are carbohydrates, and if there are any good or bad ones? How many carbs should we have every day, and what are whole grain fibers? Will eating carbs increase my weight? EAT GOOD or DIE BAD will discuss all this and a lot more about carbohydrates in the following section.

So what are carbohydrates?

Carbohydrates are the naturally occurring sugars, fiber, and starches in food. All of the carbs are made up of these sugar molecules linked together to form fiber and starches. In the body, sugars and starches break down in eth digestive system to form glucose. Glucose is the primary fuel that gives energy and powers all of the body functions. Glucose is also known as blood sugar. Dietary fiber is the kind of carbs that are not broken in the digestion process. It goes through the stomach, small intestine, colon and is then discarded out of the body.

Dieticians and scientists form grouping or carbs in two main types: i.e., complex carbs and simple carbs. Complex carbs are the fiber and starches. Simple carbs are the sugars that occur naturally in vegetables, fruits, milk, brown sugar, honey, white sugar, and other food processing. In the current days, carbs are classified based on their ingredients and fiber content.

What are good and bad carbs?

These are the terms that most diet promoters have made famous. Usually, good carbs are foods that contain high fiber amounts. These carbs take a lot longer to break down in the body and are used for energy. They are mostly found in whole grain bread and certain cereals, vegetables, whole wheat flour, and fruits. Bad carbs are the foods that have refined carbs with lower amounts of fiber, which are mainly white flour and sugar. These are present in foods like cakes, cookies, white bread, and other items from the bakery made of white flour, white rice, and a few cereal bowls.

Dividing the carbs into good and bad carbs is just an easy way to think about nutrition, but these aren't exactly scientific terms. When you want to eat a healthy diet, pick a high fiber, whole grain food rather than having low fiber ones.

How many carbohydrates do I need in a day?

Instead of just counting the carbs, dieticians are recommending planning the meals using a Healthy Plate. Half of your plate must fill with vegetables and fruits on each meal and fill a quarter of it with whole grains. Potatoes and French fries are not considered healthy vegetables by scientists. The last quarter left on the plate must be meat, beans, fish, or nuts.

Why should you have whole grains?

Whole grains are the ideal source of having carbs in your body as they give you energy and minerals, vitamins, and fiber. Eating whole grains mostly instead of consuming highly refined grains such as white flour and white rice may help reduce the risk of developing heart disease and diabetes. It will also keep your digestive system healthy. Foods that are made from whole grains can give you high fiber content.

Why should I have high amounts of fiber?

Fiber is mostly found in vegetables, legumes, fruits, and whole grains. Fiber gives a healthy digestive system as it keeps the bowels moving. It may also help prevent obesity development in the body and the risk of heart diseases and diabetes as it slows down the process of digestion and keeps you feeling full for long. Fiber may be soluble and dissolve in water or be insoluble and not dissolve in water. Soluble fiber may be found in many fruits and a few vegetables, including peas, corn, carrots, oatmeal, nuts, dry beans, and seeds. When they are mixed with water indigestion, these fibers become thick and gelatin material kind. Soluble fiber may also help lower cholesterol levels and blood glucose.

Insoluble fibers are found in many kinds of foods, especially foods made of whole wheat flour, brown rice, whole grain cereals, many vegetables, and fruits. Insoluble fibers assist the body in moving the waste in the digestive system. It can also help in the prevention of tiny blood clots that may cause heart attacks and strokes.

Carbs are essential in helping our bodies maintain their natural functions. It would help if you had the right amounts of carbs in your daily life so that your body can usually work.

Protein

Dietary proteins are among the most important topics when the concern is your physique and improvements in it. If you have ever thought about what proteins are and why they are so important or how much you must be eating, this section of the guide EAT GOOD or DIE BAD can help you build a sound understanding.

What are Proteins?

Proteins are the organic molecules made of amino acids that are the building blocks of life. These amino acids are linked together by chemical bonds. They are then folded in many different ways to create the three-dimensional structures important to our body's functions.

There are at first two main kinds of amino acids in our body. First, we have the essential amino acids that the body cannot produce or manufacture, and hence we have to obtain them through our diets. A few amino acids are conditionally essential. It means that our bodies won't always make them as much as we need. Situations of stress can inhibit their production levels. Next are the nonessential amino acids, the ones that our bodies can naturally produce.

Examples of three kinds of amino acids:

Essential amino acids

Histidine

Isoleucine

Lysine

Methionine

Threonine

Valine

Tryptophan

Conditionally essential amino acids

Arginine

Cysteine

Glutamine

Tyrosine

Nonessential amino acids

Alanine

Asparagine's

Aspartic acid

Glutamic acid

Proline

Serine

Why is it important to have proteins?

During digestion, the body breaks the protein we eat to form individual amino acids contributing to the plasma pool of these amino acids. This pool is the storage reserve of amino acids that circulate in the body through blood. The amino acid pool present in the bloodstream readily trades with amino acids. The cells' proteins give a supply of amino acids just as needed and are also continuously replenished. Since the bodies require amino acids and proteins to produce many essential molecules in the body such as hormones, enzymes, antibodies, and neurotransmitters, this happens without protein intake. Our bodies won't be able to function well.

Protein lets our bodies replace the old cells, transport many substances in the body, and help repair and grow them. Consuming protein may also increase glucagon hormone levels, which helps in eth control of body fat. Glucagon is then released in the body when the levels of blood sugar dropdown. Protein makes the liver break down the stored glycogen into glucose so that body can use it. It may also help in the liberation of free fatty acids from the adipose tissue, which is another way to get the right fuel for cells. Protein makes the body fat be used somewhere usefully instead of hanging on the body midsection.

How much protein should I take?

How much protein you should take depends on a few factors, but the one main one is the activity level. The primary suggestion for protein intake is only .8 grams per kilogram of body mass in an untrained and generally healthy adult. For example, a 150 lbs. man would have around 45 grams every day. But this amount is only to keep protein deficiency away. It is not necessary and optimal, especially for people who are athletes that train hard every day. For people who are doing high-intensity training, protein needs rise higher to 1.2 to 2.0 g/kg of the whole-body mass. Hence a man of 150 lbs. will require 95 to 135 protein every day.

Can I have too much protein?

If you have an issue with overeating protein, the extra protein may convert into fat or sugar in your body.

However, protein isn't as quickly or easily turned into fat or carbs as the thermic effect is very high on protein than fat and carbs. While 30% of the energy of protein goes into digestion, absorption, and in the process of assimilation, only 8% of life from carbs and 3% of energy from fats do the same.

Having higher protein levels may help you feel full for longer and can keep your tummy filling full. You won't be going into the kitchen again and again to have more food.

Fats

When people are talking about fats, they often call them bad. Some of this is just because a few types of fats and also the fat-like substance called cholesterol may be the culprit for giving you the following:

- Diabetes

- Cancer

- Obesity

- Cardiovascular disease

But all of these fats aren't equal. A few fats are good for you than a few others and can also give you sound health. Knowing the difference between them can help you make sure which of the fats you need to stay away from and which one of them you can eat in balanced amounts. Research is still evolving on dietary fat, but a few facts are already apparent. Dietary fat, known as fatty acids, may be found in foods obtained from animals and plants. Certain fats may have been linked to adverse effects on our heart's health, but the rest are found to give many essential health benefits.

Fat is essential for your diet, just as protein and carbs keep your body fueled up with energy. Certain body functions also heavily rely on the presence of fat in our diet and body. For example, a few vitamins need fat to dissolve in the bloodstream and give you nutrients. However, the abundance of calories from having a lot of fat of any kind may lead to a significant gain in weight. Foods and oils have a mix of fatty acids, but the dominant type of fat they have is what makes them healthy or not healthy.

Which are the less healthy fats?

Two kinds of fats that include trans-fat and saturated fat, have already been identified as harmful to human health. Many of the foods that have these kinds of fats are solid at room temperature, such as the following:

- Margarine

- Butter

- Shortening

- Beef or pork fat

Trans fat must be avoided, whereas you must eat saturated fat.

Saturated fats must eat sparingly

Most of the saturated fats are animal fats. They are observed in high amounts in dairy products and fatty meats.

The sources of saturated fats include:

- Dark chicken meat and poultry skin

- Fatty cuts of pork, beef, and lamb

- High-fat dairy items

- Tropical oils

- Lard

Having too much-saturated fats may also increase blood cholesterol levels and even lousy cholesterol levels. Traditional doctors have connected higher saturated fats consumption with the increase of heart diseases.

Trans fats are to be avoided when possible.

Short of trans fatty acids that are trans-fat appear in foods that have partially hydrogenated vegetable oils. These are the worst kind of fats for you.

You may find trans-fat in the following:

- Fried food items such as fries, deep-fried fast foods, doughnuts

- Margarine

- Vegetable shortening

- Baked goods

- Processed snack foods

Like trans-fat, saturated fats can raise the LDL in your blood and are also known as bad cholesterol. Trans fat may also suppress the good cholesterol in your body. Doctors have linked trans-fat to cause an increase in the risk of inflammation in our bodies. This inflammation may also cause harmful effects on our health. These health effects include diabetes, heart disease, and stroke. A few margarine kinds may have trans fats in them if made with hydrogenated ingredients; hence it must be made sure that you are choosing non-hydrogenated versions.

Foods that have good fats

Doctors have considered monosaturated fats and poly saturated fats as healthier for our hearts. These are the fats that are a better option for your diet. Foods that have these healthy fats have to be liquid when they are left at room temperature. An example is vegetable oil. Monosaturated type fats are present in many kinds of foods and oils. The following foods have high amounts of them:

- Nuts
- Vegetable oils
- Peanut butter
- Avocado

Many types of research have proved that fats are better than being bad for our health. While trans fats are harmful to our health, saturated fats are not linked to increased heart disease risk. They likely are not as healthy as the monosaturated and poly saturated fats may be.

Dietary Fiber

Choosing tasty foods that are full of fiber as well isn't a comfortable ride. You have to find out how much dietary fiber your body needs, which foods have this fiber, and how you can add them to your meals and snacks.

So, what are dietary fibers?

Dietary fiber is also known as bulk or roughage. It is included in the parts of plant foods that your body can not absorb or digest. Unlike many other food components, like the proteins, fats, or carbohydrates that the body breaks down or fascinates, fiber is not digested by the body. Instead, it goes intact through the body, passing from the stomach, small intestine, and colon and then out of the body. Fiber is primarily categorized as soluble, dissolving in water, or insoluble, which doesn't dissolve.

Soluble Fiber: This kind of fiber dissolves in water to create a gel-like material. It can help lower blood cholesterol and also levels of glucose. Soluble fibers are found in peas, oats, beans, citrus fruits, apples, barley, and psyllium.

Insoluble Fiber: This is the type of fiber that promotes the movement of material into your digestive system and increases the stool bulk to benefit those who struggle with having a stool or have an issue of constipation. Whole wheat flour, nuts, wheat bran, beans, and vegetables have this fiber type. The amount of soluble or insoluble fibers greatly varies in many different plants. To receive the most health benefits, you must eat a wide variety of high-fiber foods.

What are the benefits of having a high-fiber diet?

A high fiber diet can help you in the following ways:

Normalize bowel movements

Dietary fibers help in increasing the size and weight of the stool and also softens it. A bulky stool is comparatively easier to pass; it decreases the chances of constipation. If you have loose and watery stools, then fiber may help solidify your stool as it absorbs water and adds to the bulk of the stool.

Helps maintain bowel health

A high fiber diet can lower your risk of having hemorrhoids and also small pouches in the colon. Studies have also found out that high fiber diets can reduce the chances of developing colorectal cancer. A few fibers are fermented in the colon. Researchers are looking at how this might play a role in the prevention of diseases of the colon.

Lowers cholesterol levels

Soluble fiber found in oats, beans, flaxseed, and oat bran might lower the total blood cholesterol levels by lowering the low-density lipoprotein or the harmful cholesterol levels. Studies have revealed that high fiber foods might have many heart health benefits, including reducing inflammation and blood pressure.

Helps control blood sugar levels

In people who have diabetes, fiber, especially soluble fiber, can slow down sugar absorption and improve blood sugar levels. Healthy diets that include insoluble fiber may also reduce the risk of having type 2 diabetes.

Aids in acquiring an ideal weight

High fiber foods are more filling than low fiber foods; hence, you are more likely to eat a lot less and stay satisfied. High fiber foods also take longer to be eaten and are also less energy-dense, which means they have fewer calories in the same food volume.

Helps you live a lot longer

Many studies have suggested that dietary fiber intake reduces the risk of dying from cancers and all cardiovascular disease.

How much fiber should I take?

Researches have provided many sciences and fact-based advice on matters of health and medicine. According to these researches, the following is a dietary fiber that one should take being an adult.

Ages 50 or younger:

Men should take 38 grams per day

Women should take 25 grams per day

Age 51 or older:

Men should take 30 grams per day

Women should take 21 grams per day

You can take the most dietary fiber from the following options:

Whole grain products

Fruits

Vegetables

Nuts and seeds

Peas, beans, and other legumes

Having dietary fiber added to your daily food choices will help improve your quality of life.

Vitamins

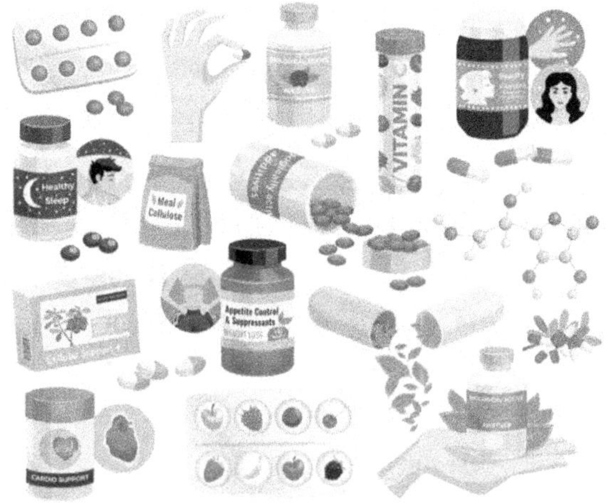

Vitamins are organic compounds that are needed in small quantities. Most of the vitamins need to be obtained from food sources as our body cannot produce them or can do it in tiny amounts. Each organism has different needs for vitamins. For example, humans need to have vitamin C through their diets, whereas dogs can produce vitamin C in their bodies. For humans, vitamin D is not readily available in considerable quantities in food. The human body then synthesizes this vitamin when exposed to sunlight, and hence this is the ideal source of vitamin D for our bodies.

Many various vitamins play different vital roles in the body, and every person needs an additional amount of every vitamin to remain healthy. Through this section of this guide, you will get to know what vitamins are, what their role is in our body, and through which foods you can obtain the most of it.

What are vitamins?

Vitamins are those organic substances that are present in small amounts in natural foodstuffs. Having tiny amounts of any vitamin may increase the risk of having certain illnesses and health issues. A vitamin is an organic compound that means it has carbon in it. It is also an essential nutrient in the body that you may need to obtain from food. The following are the types of vitamins:

Fat-soluble and water-soluble vitamins

Vitamins are either soluble or dissolvable in water or fat. Both of these types are described below:

Fat-soluble vitamins

Vitamins such as A, D, E, and K are fat-soluble vitamins. The body keeps storage of fat-soluble vitamins in the liver and fatty tissue, and the stores of these vitamins can also stay in the body for many days and months. Dietary fats let the body absorb these vitamins through the intestinal tract.

Water-soluble vitamins

Water-soluble vitamins do not remain in the body for long, and they cannot also be stored. They leave the body through urine. Thus, people need to have a more constant and regular supply of water-soluble vitamins than fat-soluble ones. Vitamin C and all of the B vitamins are water-soluble.

The 13 types of vitamins are listed as below:

Vitamin A: Helps with improving eye health

Vitamin B1: It is essential for producing certain enzymes that help in the breakdown of sugar

Vitamin B2: it is necessary for the growth and the development of cells in our body and helps metabolize food.

Vitamin B3: The body requires niacin for our cells to grow and work properly.

Vitamin B5: It is needed to produce the right amount of energy hormones.

Vitamin B6: It is essential for the proper formation of red blood cells.

Vitamin B7: It lets the body metabolize fats, proteins, and carbs. It also contributes to keratin, a structural protein present in nails, hair, and skin.

Vitamin B9: It is essential for the formation of DNA and RNA

Vitamin B12: It is necessary to maintain a healthy nervous system.

Vitamin C: It contributes to the production of collagen, wound healing, and also in bone formation. It improves the strength of blood vessels, supports our immune system and helps the body to be able to absorb iron, and also acts as an excellent antioxidant.

Vitamin D: It is essential to give healthy mineralization to the bone

Vitamin E: It has antioxidant activity that helps prevent oxidative stress, which is an issue that increases the risk of many inflammation and other diseases.

Vitamin K: It is essential for blood clotting.

Vitamin Supplements

Most people in the US take multivitamins and many other supplements. Research says that this may not be helpful or necessary. A balanced and varied diet with many fruits and vegetables must be the primary source of vitamins. Fortified foods and specific supplements might be appropriate in a few cases; however, just like in pregnancy, people with restricted diets and particular health issues.

Anyone taking supplements must also be careful not to exceed the maximum dose you can have. Having too much vitamin may lead to health issues. Also, a few medications may interact with vitamin supplements as well.

Minerals

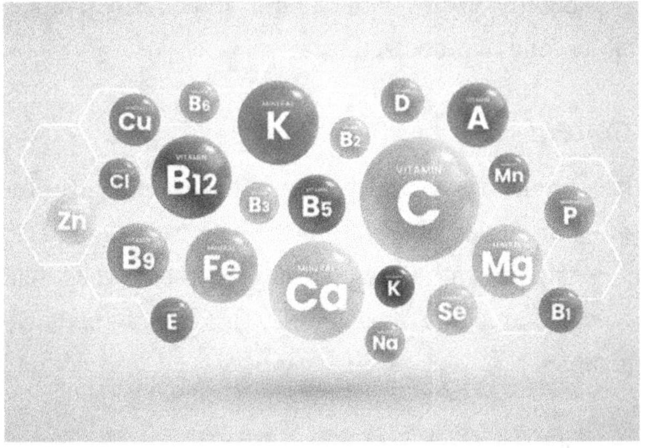

Our body needs many kinds of minerals; these are named as the essential minerals. Essential minerals are mainly divided into many various minerals, i.e., major minerals and trace minerals. These two groups of minerals are just equally important, but the trace minerals are needed in a lot lesser amounts compared to the major ones. The parts required in our bodies are not an indication of the importance of these minerals.

A balanced diet mostly gives you all the essential minerals. There are certain kinds of minerals, most of which are given below and the function they perform.

Sodium

It is needed for maintaining a proper fluid balance, muscle contraction, and nerve transmission. You can obtain sodium from table salt, milk, soy sauce, vegetables, and unprocessed meat.

Chloride

It is needed for a proper balance of fluid and also for stomach acid. It can obtain from soy sauce and table salt, which is significantly present in processed foods that include small amounts of such milk. Bread, meat and also in vegetables.

Potassium

It is needed for fluid balance and also for nerve transmission. The source foods for this mineral are milk, meats, fruits, whole grains, and legumes.

Calcium

It is essential for teeth and bone health; it helps in relaxing the muscles and their contraction. It is necessary for the nerve's functioning, blood pressure regulation, and nerve functioning. It regulates immune system health. You can obtain this mineral from milk and products made of milk.

Phosphorus

It is essential to keep healthy teeth and bones; it is found in each of your cells and is a part of the system that supports the acid-base balance. It can obtain from fish, meat, poultry, processed foods.

Magnesium

It is found in bones and is needed to make protein, nerve transmission, muscle contraction, and immune system health. It can obtain from nuts and seeds, leafy green vegetables, and seafood.

Sulfur

It is found in protein muscles and can be obtained from foods like meats, fish, eggs and legumes, and nuts.

What are the Minerals in foods?

Minerals are needed for us to do the three main things as follows:

- Build strong teeth
- Control body fluids within and outside cells

- Turn the food we consume into energy.

Which foods have Minerals in them?

Minerals are present in foods like bread, cereals, fish, meat, dairy, milk, nuts, fruits, and vegetables. We need to have more minerals than a few others. We need to have some minerals that can help us regulate our body's functions and live a high quality of life. Minerals like calcium, phosphorus, sodium, magnesium, potassium, and chloride are needed in higher amounts than iron, iodine, zinc, copper, and selenium.

Trace minerals are needed to maintain many functions for our body, such as boost energy metabolism; they make protein and the human body's genetic material. These minerals help our bodies to carry out the normal functioning of many natural processes. These are parts of the enzyme and are there in eth formation of teeth and bones. They are also present in some enzymes.

Your body requires an adequate amount of minerals so that your teeth and bones can remain healthy and strong, and the food you eat can convert to energy efficiency. And with vitamins, having a healthy and balanced diet must provide all the minerals that your body needs to function correctly. Most of the essential minerals include iron, calcium, and potassium.

Minerals are obtained from various sources, but the most efficient source is to get them from food options. You can also take supplements and fulfill the deficiency of minerals caused in your body for various reasons. Having the right amount of minerals in your body will help you grow, stay healthy, and develop rightly. The body utilizes minerals to carry out various functions, such as building strong bones and transmitting nerve impulses. A few minerals are also used to make hormones and also maintain a regular heartbeat.

The best way to have minerals in your daily life is to obtain them from your diet, as this will not cause any of the side effects for you. You can maintain your body and all its functions by giving it all that it needs to function perfectly. These are the essential minerals for your body as they help you grow properly and live a quality life. You can significantly improve your quality of life by maintaining your diet and also your exercise option.

Part 2

NUTRITION & HUMAN BODY

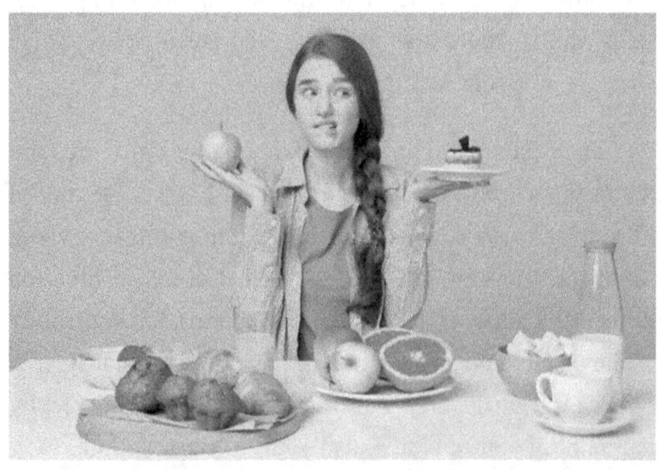

The human body is mainly composed of the thoughts our minds create, the things we do, and the DIET that we eat. All these three factors contribute to our well-being and make us who we are. Whatever diet you take affects your body systems and parts in different ways. Hence some diets affect your brain, your heart, and other parts of your body. This section will all be about specific diets for various body functions and features.

1. Brain Diet: Nourishing, Protecting, and Enhancing Brain Power by using Healthy Food.

2. Heart Diet: Healthy Food for Protecting Heart.

3. Lungs Diet: Nutritious Food to Support and Protect Lungs.

4. Stomach Diet: Healthy Food for better Functioning of 24/7 Food Factory.

5. Kidneys Diet: Best Healthy Diet for Protecting and Normal working of Kidney.

6. Muscular Tissue: Nutrition for Muscle Cell Function.

7. Bones: Nutritious Diet for Building and Maintaining Strong Bones.

Brain Diet

The human brain is an essential part of one's body. It controls your actions and is your CPU. It would help if you kept it healthy and active to lead your daily life. But what are the essential food items that you must have so that your brain remains healthy and keeps supporting your ups and downs in life, and you can keep your memory active for long as well? So what are some of the most nutritious diets for your brain?

Fatty Fish

When people are talking about food for the brain, fatty fish is mostly a top option. Fatty fish is the type of fish that includes trout, salmon, and sardines. All of these are rich sources of omega-three fatty acids. Around 60% of our brains are made up of fat, and half of this fat is the omega 3 type. Your brain utilizes omega 3 to build the nerve and brain cells, and these fats are essential for memory and learning.

Coffee

If coffee is the main thing you consume every morning, you will be delighted to hear that it is excellent for you. Two of the main components of coffee are caffeine, and the antioxidants help your brain function better. Caffeine present in coffee has many positive effects on our brain. These effects include increased alertness, improved mood, sharpened concentration, etc. Having coffee at long times is also linked to reducing neurological diseases that Alzheimer's and Parkinson's'. Coffee is mainly because coffee has high amounts of antioxidants.

Blueberries

Blueberries give your brain many great health benefits, including a few that are good for your brain. Blueberries and also other berries give anthocyanins that are a plant compound having anti-inflammatory and also antioxidant effects. These help you with oxidative stress. A few of the antioxidants in blueberries are found to collect up in the brain and improve brain cells' communication.

Turmeric

Turmeric has created a lot of buzzes recently. This intense yellow spice is the main ingredient in many curries. It has many benefits for the brain as well. Curcumin is the active substance in turmeric, which has been shown to cross the blood and brain barrier, which may directly enter the brain and affect its cells. It is a potent antioxidant and also has anti-inflammatory properties, which have been linked to benefits like a good memory, ease in depression, and growth of new brain cells.

Brain foods can help you in Nourishing, Protecting, and Enhancing Brain Power and let you keep your memory afresh for long.

Heart Diet: Healthy Food For Protecting Heart

Out of all the diseases that happen, around one-third of them are caused due to heart diseases. Diet always plays a significant role in maintaining our heart health and may also impact heart illness risk. A few foods may even influence triglycerides, blood pressure, inflammation, and cholesterol levels, all of which are risk factors for our heart. But what are the diets that can keep our hearts strengthened and active?

Let us find out the top food items that you can take to keep your heart healthy.

Leafy Green Veggies

Leafy green veggies such as kale, spinach, and collard greens are exceptionally known to give an abundance of minerals, vitamins, and antioxidants. In particular, they are a significant vitamin K source that helps protect arteries and give you proper blood clotting. These leafy green vegetables are great to promote the health of your heart and boost the strength of your veins and arteries.

Whole Grains

Whole grains include many nutrient-rich parts of the grains, such as the germ, bran, and endosperm. Many common types of whole grains include brown rice, whole wheat, oats, quinoa, and buckwheat. Many studies have found that adding more whole grains to your diet can benefit heart health.

Berries

Strawberries, blackberries, blueberries, and raspberries are fully packed with many essential nutrients that play a vital role in maintaining your heart health. Berries are also significantly present in antioxidants that protect against oxidative stress and even inflammation. Many studies have shown that adding berries to your daily diet can reduce risk factors that cause heart diseases.

Avocados

Avocados are just an excellent source of monosaturated fats that are healthy for our hearts. These have been linked to reducing levels of cholesterol and also heart illnesses. A study revealed the effects of the three cholesterol-lowering diets among 45 overweight people with a test group consuming an avocado per day. The avocados groups showed a reduction in the bad cholesterol, including lower levels of small and dense LDL. Avocados are just great for reducing your cholesterol, blood pressure, and the risk of having metabolic syndrome.

Fatty fish and fish oil

Fatty fish, including sardines, tuna, and salmon, are full of omega 3 fatty acids. These have been proven to be great for our hearts. If you do not consume that much seafood, having fish oil is just a great option to get your daily dose of omega 3 fatty acids. Heart-healthy food items can boost your longevity.

lungs diet: nutritious food to support and protect lungs

Your lungs need to be functioning correctly and with strength so that you can live life at its best. Keeping the lungs healthy is very important. Many everyday factors can harm our lung health, which includes exposure to cigarette smoke and environmental toxins. The following diets can help you maintain your lung health.

Beets and Beet Greens

This vibrantly colored root and the greens of the beetroot plant have compounds that optimize lung function. Beetroot and beet greens are dense with nitrates. These have been shown to benefit lung function. Nitrates can help relax your vessels, reduce blood pressure and optimize oxygen uptake. Beetroot supplements are seen to improve physical performance and also lung function among people having lung conditions.

Peppers

Peppers are among the richest sources of Vitamin C, a water-soluble nutrient that also acts as an excellent antioxidant in your body. Having enough vitamin C is very important for people who are used to smoking. Consuming a single medium-size sweet red pepper may deliver 169% of the suggested intake of vitamin C.

Apples

According to research, eating apples daily can help with lung function. Studies have also shown that apple intake is linked to a slow decline of lung function for people who have quit smoking. Having five or more apples a week is linked with better lung function and reduced COPD risk. Apple intake can also reduce your risk of asthma and even lung cancer.

Pumpkin

The very brightly colored flesh of these giant vegetables has a variety of lung-benefiting plant compounds. They are also rich in carotenoids, which include lutein, carotene, and zeaxanthin. Studies have revealed that higher blood levels of carotenoids are linked with proper functioning in young and older people.

Turmeric

Turmeric is mainly used to give many overall health benefits as it has many anti-inflammatory and antioxidant properties. Curcumin, which is the main element in turmeric, might greatly support your lung function. A higher intake of curcumin is linked with 9.2% of better lung function than smokers who did not have curcumin.

Having healthy lung diets will improve your lungs' function and benefit you, especially in your more senior years. These diets have helped ex-smokers regain their lungs' health and come back from the harm that happened to them due to smoking.

Stomach Diet: Healthy Food For Better Functioning Of 24/7 Food Factory

Whatever we eat significantly affects our body, but the first thing it affects is the stomach. Our diet options can intensely turn down or turn up the health of our stomach. You may see so many changes in your body only by changing what you eat. So let us find out what are food choices that can improve the health of your stomach.

Yogurt

Yogurt is made of milk that has been fermented due to the lactic acid bacteria. It has friendly bacteria called probiotics that are great for bacteria that live in our digestive tract. It can help improve digestion and also keeps your gut healthy. In contrast, probiotics can naturally be there in your gut by having foods that contain them. Yogurt is abundant in probiotics and can help with digestive issues, constipation, and bloating. When you shop for yogurts, make sure you look for the ones with titled live and active cultures.

Apples

Apples are a rich source of a soluble fiber called pectin. Pectin goes through digestion in the small intestine and is then broken into the friendly bacteria present in your colon. It also increases the volume of your stool and is also commonly used to solve diarrhea and constipation. It is also shown to reduce the risk of many intestinal infections and even inflammation in the colon.

Fennel

Fennel is a plant with long green stalks with a pale bulb and adds flavor to your food. It is the fiber content that keeps constipation away and also improves the regularity in your digestive tract. Fennel also has the antispasmodic agent, which relaxes the smooth muscles in the digestive tract.

Kefir

Kefir is a cultured dairy product that is made by the addition of kefir grains into milk. These grains result in the mixing of bacteria and yeast with milk and appear to give digestive benefits. Like the probiotics in yogurt, kefir has a culture that aids the digestion of lactose. It decreases some of the adverse side effects of lactose intolerance, such as cramping, gas, and bloating. Kefir has been linked to reducing inflammation in the gut, which further improves the digestion process.

Chia Seeds

Chia seeds are a great source of fiber, which causes them to take the form of gelatin kind substance in the stomach once they are consumed. They act like the probiotic, which supports healthy bacteria's growth in the gut and contributes to healthy digestion.

These healthy stomach diets are straightforward to consume and help you stay more active in your life. You can obtain the best of your life by eating healthy.

Kidneys Diet

Best Healthy Diet for Protecting and Normal working of Kidneys are tiny organs in the lower abdomen, which play an essential role in our bodies' health. A few foods might boost our kidneys' performance, whereas others may put stress on their working and may also cause damage. Hence let us find out the best diets that can improve the working of our kidneys.

Water:

Water is the best beverage that you may have at any time of the day. It is best for all the body functions and should not be taken any less than maximum. Our cells utilize water to transport certain toxins into our blood. The kidneys use water to filter out these toxins and make urine, which transports them out of our bodies. All of these healthy actions can do by having an adequate amount of water intake.

Fatty Fish:

Salmon, tuna, and much other cold water, fatty fish that are very high in omega 3 fatty acids may make a healthy addition to any of your diets. The body may not make enough omega 3 fatty acids that mean that you have to obtain them from your diet. Fatty fish is just an ideal source of having these healthy fats. Omega fats may also help reduce the fat levels in the blood and slightly reduce the blood pressure. As high blood pressure is a significant risk factor for kidney illness, looking for a way to lower it might protect your kidneys.

Sweet Potatoes

Sweet potatoes are just the same as white potatoes, but they have an excess of fiber, which may cause them to break a lot slower—coffee results in a reduced spike in insulin levels. Sweet potatoes also have vitamins and minerals such as potassium, which can help balance sodium levels present in the body and reduce its results on kidneys.

Dark Leafy Greens

Dark leafy greens that include kale, spinach, and chard are great dietary staples with many fibers, vitamins, and minerals. Many of them also have protective compounds, which include antioxidants. However, these foods are higher in potassium, so they might not be suitable for a restricted diet or dialysis.

Berries

Dark berries also include blueberries, strawberries, and raspberries, which are a great source of the most helpful nutrients and antioxidant compounds. These might also help in the protection of cells in the body against any damage. Berries are very likely to have a better option than most sugary foods to satisfy a sweet craving.

Muscular Tissue: Nutrition For Muscle Cell Function

Having a lot of physical activity and eating the right foods is very important to maintain muscle health. You need to be actively involved in eating the suitable food options and how your muscles. Let us determine which foods are good for maintaining your muscles' health and giving the right amount of nutrition to the muscle cell functions.

Eggs

Eggs have high-quality protein, healthy fats, and many other nutrients, such as the other necessary nutrients such as B vitamins and choline. Proteins are made of amino acids and eggs with vast amounts of amino acids that are important for muscle growth. Also, B vitamins are essential for our bodies' processes, including high energy production.

Salmon

Salmon is a very healthy choice for building your muscles and also for your overall health. Every 3-ounce serving of salmon has around 17 grams of protein and almost 2 grams of omega 3 fatty acids, and many essential B vitamins. Omega 3 fatty acids also play a vital role in muscular health and increase muscle gain while exercising.

Chicken Breast

There are excellent reasons why chicken breasts are thought of as a staple for gaining muscle. They are full of protein with every 3-ounce serving, which has around 26 grams of good quality protein. They also have a good amount of B vitamins B6 and Niacin that may be specifically important if you are physically active. These vitamins can help your body work properly while you are in physical activity and exercise, which is essential for optimal muscle gain. A few research types have also shown that diets with higher protein may also help in fat loss.

Greek Yogurt

Dairy has very high-quality protein and a mixture of very fast-digesting whey protein and even the slow-digesting casein protein. A few research types have shown that people also experience increased lean mass when combining the fast and slow-digesting dairy proteins. But not all dairy is formed as equal. Greek yogurt may have approximately double the number of proteins as regular yogurt. While Greek yogurt is an ideal snack to have at any time, eating it right after your workout session or before bed may be significant as it has a mixture of fast and slow-digesting proteins.

These are a few diet choices that can help you boost your muscles and gain the best muscle strength.

Bones: Nutritious Diet For Building And Maintaining Strong Bones

You want to have strong bones so that you do not end up breaking any of them while you are out in your life. It would help if you had a lot of strength in your bones, which can best achieve a good diet. Which diet choices can help you have the best power in your bones? Well, let's find out.

Vegetables

Having a lot of vegetables is the best suggestion we have for you to gain more robust bones. They are one of the ideal sources of vitamin C that stimulates the production of cells forming bones. A few studies also suggest that vitamin C antioxidant effects might also protect the bones from damage. Vegetables also seem to have a good bone mineral density increase, known as bone density. Bone density calculates Calcium's number and all of the other minerals present in your bones.

High Protein Diet

Getting a lot of protein is essential for your healthy and strong bones. 50% of your bone is made up of protein, and you must give your bones a stable supply of protein so that they can stay strong. But make sure you do not have a lot of protein as that may cause a leach of Calcium in the bones so that you will have more acidity in your blood.

Have High Calcium Foods

Calcium is one of the essential minerals for your bone health, and it is also the primary mineral present in your bones. Because the old bone cells are breaking down constantly and are replaced by the newer ones, it is essential to have a steady intake of Calcium to protect the bone structure and its strength.

These are the best diets you may have to support the strength of your bones. Have them and have healthy bones in later years of your life as well.

Part 3

HEALTHY EATING PLANS FOR DIFFERENT AGE GROUPS

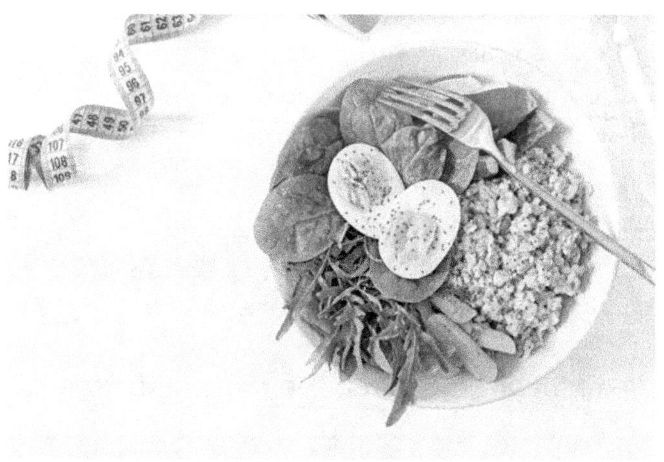

Not all can eat, all right? Your age majorly defines what your body needs are and what kind of diets you should be eating at which age. With the years growing on your life calendar, your physical and dietary requirements will keep changing. Hence let's get introduced to different healthy eating plans that would help you be the best version of yourself at any age.

1. Nutrition and Diet Plan for Kids.

2. Nutrition and Diet Plan for Women.

3. Nutrition and Diet Plan for Men.

Nutrition And Diet Plan For Kids

Nutrition for kids is mainly based on the same kinds of principles as that for adults. Everyone needs a similar type of food, including minerals, vitamins, carbohydrates, fat, and protein. Children, however, have to go with different amounts of all these nutrients at different ages. So, which can be the best way to fuel the child's growth and also their development? The following section of this guide will help you pick up the ideal diet choices for your kids. These are based on medical facts; hence you can rely on them straight away.

The following diets must be there in the foods:

Protein: Choose seafood, poultry, and lean meat along with eggs, poultry, peas, beans, soy products, and seeds or unsalted nuts. These items have high amounts of protein in them that are essential for your kid's body's healthy development.

Fruits: Encourage your kids to eat many fresh, canned, dried, or frozen fruits rather than forcing fruit juice on them. If your child takes a lot of fruit juice, make sure it is wholly and entirely juice without any added sugars, and you should also limit his/her servings. Look out for canned fruit that says it is light or is packed in its juice, which means it is lower in added sugar. Keep in mind that a quarter cup of dried fruit equals only a cup equivalent of fruit. When it is consumed in excess, dried fruits may contribute to the extra calories.

Vegetables: Serve many kinds of fresh, frozen, canned, or dried vegetables to your kids. Aim to provide various types of vegetables, including dark green, orange, red beans and peas, starchy, and many other types of vegetables every week. When you are selecting frozen or canned vegetables, make sure you look out for low sodium options.

Grains: Choose whole grains, including whole grains wheat bread, popcorn, oatmeal, quinoa, and brown or wild rice. Limit having refined grains like pasta, white bread, and rice.

Dairy: Encourage your kids to eat or drink low-fat or fat-free dairy products. These must include milk, yogurt, fortified soy beverages, or cheese.

__Make sure you limit the following food options from your kid's diet:__

Added sugar: Limit any added sugar in your kids' diet. Naturally occurring sugars that include fruit and milk are not what added sugars are; examples of added sugars are brown sugar, corn syrup, corn sweetener, honey, and others. Also, check out for nutrition labels. Choose the cereals that have minimal added sugars. Avoid any drinks that have added sugars, which include soda and energy drinks.

Saturated and trans-fat: Limit saturated fats, which are the ones that come mainly from animal sources of food, which include red meat, full-fat dairy, and poultry items. Look out for ways through which you can replace saturated fats along with nut oils and vegetables that provide you essential fatty acids and vitamin E. Healthier fats are there naturally in nuts, olives, seafood, and avocados. Limit having trans fats by not having foods that contain partially hydrogenated oil.

Sodium: Most US kids have a lot of sodium in their daily food choices. Encourage snacking on veggies and fruits instead of having cookies or chips. Check for nutrition labels and also look out for products that have low sodium levels.

If you are concerned about your kid's nutrition or have some concerns about your kid's diet, you must talk to your doctor or the registered dietician for your kid.

Daily intake for ages 2 to 4 for Girls:

- Calories: 1,000 TO 1,400 Depending on the growth and levels of activity
- Protein: 2 to 4 ounces
- Fruits: 1 to 1.5 cups
- Vegetables: 1 to 1.5 cups
- Grains: 3 to 5 ounces
- Dairy: 2 to 2.5 cups

Daily intake for ages 2 to 4 for Boys:

- Calories: 1,000 to 1,600 Depending on the growth and levels of activity
- Protein: 2 to 5 ounces
- Fruits: 1 to 1.5 cups
- Vegetables: 1 to 2 cups
- Grains: 3 to 5 ounces
- Dairy: 2 to 2.5 cups

Daily intake for ages 5 to 8 for Girls:

- Calories: 1,200 to 1,800 Depending on the growth and levels of activity
- Protein: 3 to 5 ounces
- Fruits: 1 to 1.5 cups
- Vegetables: 1.5 to 2.5 cups
- Grains: 4 to 6 ounces
- Dairy: 2.5 cups

Daily intake for ages 5 to 8 for Boys:

- Calories: 1,200 to 2000 Depending on the growth and levels of activity
- Protein: 3 to 5.5 ounces
- Fruits: 1 to 2 cups
- Vegetables: 1.5 to 2.5 cups
- Grains: 4 to 6 ounces
- Dairy: 2.5 cups

Daily intake for ages 9 to 13 for Girls:

- Calories: 1,400 to 2200 Depending on the growth and levels of activity
- Protein: 4 to 6 ounces
- Fruits: 1.5 to 2 cups
- Vegetables: 1.5 to 3 cups
- Grains: 5 to 7 ounces

- Dairy: 3 cups

Daily intake for ages 9 to 13 for Boys:

- Calories: 1,600 to 2600 Depending on the growth and levels of activity
- Protein: 5 to 6.5 ounces
- Fruits: 1.5 to 2 cups
- Vegetables: 2 to 3.5 cups
- Grains: 5 to 9 ounces
- Dairy: 3 cups

Daily intake for ages 14 to 18 for Girls:

- Calories: 1,800 to 2400 Depending on the growth and levels of activity
- Protein: 5 to 6.5 ounces
- Fruits: 1.5 to 2 cups
- Vegetables: 2 to 3.5 cups
- Grains: 6 to 8 ounces
- Dairy: 3 cups

Daily intake for ages 14 to 18 for Boys:

- Calories: 2000 to 3200 Depending on the growth and levels of activity
- Protein: 5.5 to 7 ounces
- Fruits: 2 to 2.5 cups

- Vegetables: 2.5 to 4 cups
- Grains: 6 to 10 ounces
- Dairy: 3 cups

Nutrition And Diet Plan For Women

Women have unique nutrition needs. By eating correctly at all life stages, you may control your cravings, manage the weight, boost your energy levels, and look and feel the best.

Women and eating healthy

Trying to balance the requirements of family and work or even school and cope with the media pressure to eat and look a certain way may make your life difficult. And hence maintaining a healthy diet may seem impossible. But the right food won't only improve the mood, boost your levels of energy, help you maintain an ideal weight, and support your body through many stages of a woman's life.

Being a woman many of us are mostly prone to neglecting the dietary needs our bodies have. You might feel that you are being too busy to eat good or are used to putting your family's needs before your own. Or perhaps you are trying to be consistent on an extreme diet that leaves you short of the vital nutrients and feels hungry, cranky, and even low on energy.

It is researched well also that many women neglect their nutritional needs. Nutritional studies primarily rely on making subjects who have hormone levels more stable and predictable, making irreverent results and even misleading to the women's needs. All of this can add up to a severe shortfall in your daily nutrition.

While what goes significantly for one woman may not also be that great for another. The main thing to build up your diet on your vital nutrients. Whether you are searching for improving your mood and energy, fighting off stress or PMS, enjoying a healthy pregnancy or boosting fertility, and managing many other things in your life, the following suggestions may help you get life-changing tips.

The nutritional needs are always varied based on size, age, sex, and activity; hence the following information must be sued as a guide only. This information will reveal the daily amounts recommended on an average and a moderately active adult to get a healthy, balanced diet to maintain herself rather than lose weight. The RI for fat, sugars, saturates, and salt is in maximum amounts, whereas those for carbs and proteins are the numbers that you must meet every day.

Reference intake (IR) for women:

Energy – 2000kcal

Protein – 50g

Carbohydrates – 260g

Sugar – 90g

Fat – 70g

Saturates – 20g

Salt – 6g

Perfect portions:

Numbers and the figures given are all very well, but how can you relate it with you? You can also personalize the following parts according to your needs.

Carbs that include rice, cereal, pasta, potato:

- Portion size must be your clenched fist.

Include one portion in every main meal, and make sure it fills no more than 1/4th of your plate size.

Protein such as meat, fish, poultry, pulses, tofu:

- Portion size must be the palm of your hand
- Aim to have a portion on every meal

Cheese:

- Portion size must be 2 of your thumbs

- Enjoy like a snack or as a part of your meal

Nuts and Seeds:

- Portion size should be 1 cupped hand

- Enjoy like a snack or as a part of the meal

Butter, spreads, and nut butter

- Portion size should be the tip of the thumb

- Should eat no more than 2 to 3 times every day

Savories like crisps and popcorn:

- Portion size must be 2 of the cupped hands

- Enjoy like a snack or a treat

Bakes such as flapjacks and brownies:

- Portion size must be 2 of your fingers

- Enjoy like an occasional treat

Breakfast

It would help if you kicked start your metabolism by adding protein to your breakfast. Pick from options like salmon, eggs, dairy, and lean ham. We burn many more calories while digesting protein rather than in carbs; hence, you can revive your metabolism by making a breakfast full of protein. And as protein keeps you feeling fuller for a lot longer, you will eat fewer calories during the rest of the day.

A protein breakfast should be that long to prepare. You can top your morning toast with an egg, a slice of salmon, or some lean ham, and when you have some more time, you can enjoy an omelet or a frittata. Whatever you may do, make sure you are not skipping your breakfast as it is the most important meal of your day.

Lunch

After you have a midday snack, it's time to tend towards lunch. Make a lunch that is a mix of lean protein and full of starchy carbs. Carbs-rich foods give energy, and without these, you are more likely to suffer a classic mid-afternoon craving. The key is to choose the carbs that may provide a steady boost in blood sugar, which means passing on the white sugary foods and going for the high fiber whole grains may help you manage your afternoon munchies.

Dinner

After you have your mid-afternoon snack, you may have spread. Do not curfew on carbs. They are very low on fat, rich in fiber, and help you relax during the evening. Combine them up with some healthy essential fats, just as the ones in oily fish such as salmon, sardines, mackerel, seeds, nuts, and nut oils. Your body also used these as healthy fat options and the protein overnight to have regeneration and repair for healthy skin and hair.

Nutrition And Diet Plan For Men

Food is not just to load your tummy or fuel for life. If taken right, it can help fight off diseases and also keep you feeling younger. Men should take good care of what they eat as it can significantly impact their energy levels throughout the day and their mental health.

Eating right is essential hence you must know that an ideal and healthy diet for men may include:

- At least 2 cups of fresh fruits and 2 ½ cups of veggies every day for an intake of minerals, vitamins, fiber, and photochemical.

- Whole grains should be in your diet as well. Having at least half of grains as whole grains should be your preferred choice every day.

Replace the refined grains with whole-grain cereal, bread, pasta, oats, or brown rice.

- At least 38 grams of fiber every day for young men and 30 grams of fiber every day for men above 50 years of age.

- At least give two to three servings of fish every week.

- Unsaturated fats include nuts, oils, and oil-based dressings of salads in the place of saturated fats, including full-fat dairy foods, high-fat sweets, and butter.

- 3,400 milligrams every day of potassium from vegetables, fruits, and dairy, and fish

Energy foods are also essential to be consumed

As men have an enormous muscle mass and are typically bigger than women, they need more calories throughout the day. Moderately active males require 2,200 to 2,800 calories every day. Your energy requirements greatly depend on your weight, height, and activity level. For energy and to prevent disease, men must eat whole grains that include whole-grain bread, brown rice, pasta, cereal, barley, oats, lentils, beans, vegetables, and fruits. These foods are higher in fiber content and help manage hunger and feel full and help fend off a few cancers like colon and prostate.

More than meat

Various protein foods are suggested, including seafood and many plant-based sources such as peas, beans, and soy products. Cut off on saturated fat from the high-fat meats and the full-fat dairy products and fried items. Instead, it would help if you opted for having unsaturated and heart-healthy fats that include canola, olive oil, seeds, nuts, and avocados.

Perfect portions for men:

Carbs

- Add carbs like rice, pasta, cereal, potato and make sure it is only your one clenched fist in amount

Protein:

- Add proteins like poultry, meat, tofu, fish, pulses, and portion size is only one palm of your hand

Cheese:

- Only have it as a snack or a part of your meal and keep it only 2 of your thumbs

Nuts or seeds:

- Take them only as a snack or part of the meal and keep it only as one cupped hand

Butter or spreads or nut butter:

- Take them only as only the tip of your hands

Savories such as crisps or popcorn:

- Have it only as a snack or treat and only 2 of your cupped hands

Bakes such as brownies or flapjacks:

- Take it as an occasional treat and have only 2 of your fingers

Breakfast

Whether you are headed to your office or gym as your first stop in the morning, having some protein in your breakfast is just the best way to boost your metabolism. If you exercise the first thing in the morning, then a protein-rich breakfast helps promote muscle repair and recovery. Eggs are just the best choice as they give you a strong balance in quality fat and protein. Other options are having lean meat, fish, salmon, and also some low-fat items. Protein foods are more satiating as they stay in your stomach longer.

Lunch:

After you have a light mid-day snack, now you have to get done with your lunch. Have a lunch that is a mix of starchy carbs and lean proteins. Carb-rich food options give you enough energy, and you may suffer from mid-day cramps if you miss out on them. The primary key is to pick carbs that produce a constant and steady rise in your blood sugar levels. Whole grains like whole wheat rye and can barely keep you feeling satisfied for longer durations. Rye read can keep your sugar levels steady for as long as 10 hours. Choose a sandwich that is topped with salmon, lean beef, turkey, or chicken with many salads.

Dinner

After having your mid-day snack, you can have your dinner. Don't skip out on the carbs, as they are low in fat, rich in fiber, and help you relax during the evening. Mix them up with all the essential fats that your body may use overnight for repair and regeneration. This combination is mainly necessary for having healthy hair and skin. You may quickly get these healthy fats from oily fish such as trout, salmon, mackerel and nuts, seeds, and their oils. Fill up your plate with a colorful variety of salad or vegetables or drizzle with a dressing made from rapeseed or linseed oil and add fish, meat, or beans with a proper serving of quinoa, brown rice, or the wholemeal pasta.

All these food choices are just ideal for helping you keep up with the healthiest state of your body. You may enjoy the most active and full energy lifestyle that will keep your mood better and up for all the fun that life brings. Proper food choices significantly impact our lives, and we can always benefit from them in our dark and light days. If you are enjoying a healthy lifestyle and have the right amounts of nutritional content in your diets, you will go. Otherwise, you need to update the way you have your food.

Part 4

NUTRITION, DIET & PREVENTION OF CHRONIC DISEASE

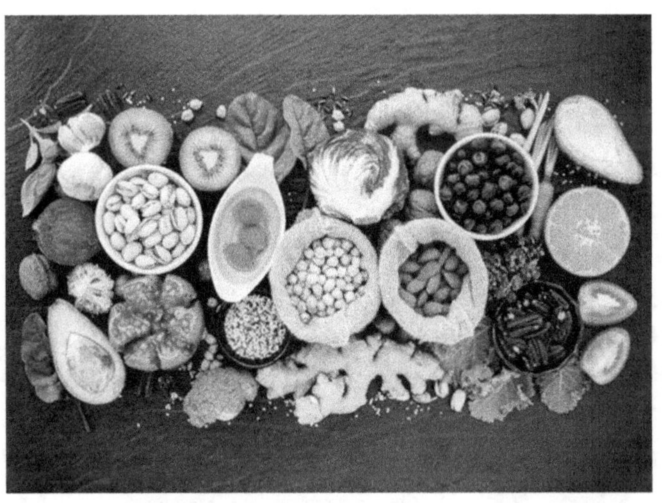

You may have known that when alarming internal rises, external help may be the lifesaver needed. Well, you may haven't heard of this, but it's true that when chronic illnesses come to bring you cloudy days, your proper diet can save you from falling, making the hole. Certain chronic illnesses that are given below can be fought well with the right kind of diet consumption.

1. Cancer

2. Heart Disease

3. Chronic Lungs Disease

4. Stroke

5. Alzheimer's

6. Diabetes

7. Kidney Disease

All chronic illnesses can well fight with the right kind of diets and nutrition to keep your body strong enough to combat such diseases. When medication doesn't work as well, the right nutrition choices can help you going strong. Let's find out which are the most common illnesses and how you can combat them with the proper food consumption.

Cancer

Cancer is the growth of malignant cells in the body that are known as tumors. Did you understand that you can stay away from the most severe chronic illnesses by having a healthy lifestyle, i.e., cancer? Research has revealed that most cancers are linked to the kind of lifestyle we adopt, including unhealthy eating patterns and a lack of physical activity. Following are a few eating tips that are best for the prevention of cancers.

Eat adequately and maintain an ideal weight

Excess body mass is linked to an increased risk of many kinds of cancers. By having an ideal and healthy body weight or losing more weight if you have an overweight BMI, you may reduce the risk. Losing weight may get complicated when you are obese, but choosing your diets wisely and having an active lifestyle may help you get back in shape.

Limit fats and added sugars

Limit having foods that have added sugars in them and solid fats that provide many calories but only a few nutrients. These foods are highly processed sugar-sweetened beverages and desserts. Calories add up with these kinds of calories dense foods very fast, leading to an increase in weight and leaving a small room for healthy, cancer-preventive foods.

Eat a lot of veggies, whole grains, and fruits

No starchy vegetables, whole grains, and whole fruits are connected with lower cancer risk. It is unclear which of the components in fruits and vegetables are the most active against carcinogenic cells. Hence enjoying many kinds of these foods as much as you can is a great way to obtain the most nutrients. Fill half of the plate with fruits and vegetables and make half of the grain's whole grains.

Moderate your portions of processed and red meat

A few studies have suggested a link between the colon and many other kinds of cancer and red meat intake. It is highly accurate for the processed meats, which include bacon, ham, and hot dogs. If you consume these kinds of foods, pick them in moderate amounts. Enjoy a small size of meat and fill up the rest of your plate with fruits, vegetables, and whole grains.

Focus on the plant proteins as well

Lentils and beans are significant sources of dietary fiber, protein, potassium, iron, and many other nutrients. Other nutrients are mostly plant-based proteins, which include tempeh and tofu. Eating many more plant proteins than animal proteins is also linked to a decreased risk of most types of cancers.

Heart Disease

Heart diseases are also very much impacted by the kind of life we live and the foods we consume. You may be impressed by how much your diet can affect the health of your heart. Many people develop heart illnesses by not having healthy diets. The following diets may be suitable for maintaining your heart health:

Leafy green vegetables

Leafy green vegetables, including kale, spinach, and collard greens, are extensively known for giving your body minerals, vitamins, and antioxidants. They are an especially great source of vitamin K that helps protect your arteries and promotes proper blood clotting. They are also high in dietary nitrates that have been shown to reduce high blood pressure and arterial stiffness and improve the cells' function in the blood vessels. A few studies have also found a strong link between increasing the intake of green vegetables and the reduced risk of heart disease.

Whole Grains

Whole grains come with all three rich in nutrient parts: the germ, endosperm, and the bran. A few common types of whole grains are brown rice, oats, barley, and whole wheat. As compared to the refined grains, whole grains are way higher in fiber that may also help reduce LDL cholesterol and reduce the risk of heart illnesses. Many studies have also found that having more whole grains in your diet may also benefit heart health.

Green Tea

Green tea has also been related to many health benefits, including burning the fat and improving insulin sensitivity. It is also brimming with catechins and polyphenols that can act as antioxidants to prevent cell damage, protect your heart health, and even reduce inflammation. According to a review, the higher intake of green tea catechins is linked to a significant decrease in LDL levels and total cholesterol. Taking green tea supplements or drinking matcha is a beverage that is a lot similar to green tea but is made with the tea leaf in it may help with heart health.

Edamame

Edamame is an immature form of soybean that is mainly used in Asian cuisine. Like other soy products, edamame is very rich in soy isoflavones, a type of flavonoid that might help decrease cholesterol levels and improve your heart health. When combined with a few changes in diet and lifestyle, a slight reduction in the cholesterol level may significantly impact heart disease risk.

Olive Oil

Mediterranean diet is just full of this oil as it gives many hearts healthy benefits. Olive oil is full of antioxidants that may relieve inflammation and decrease the risk of chronic disease. It is also rich which monosaturated fatty acids, and many studies have been linked with the improvements in health that olive oil shows. A higher intake of olive oil is connected to a 48% reduced risk of dying due to heart disease. Another extensive study has shown that higher olive oil information is linked to reduced systolic and diastolic BP. You may drizzle some olive oil on top of your cooked dishes or add it to sauces as well.

Chronic Lungs Disease

People who have developed chronic lung illness are often told that they must improve their diet choices. Not following bad eating habits may help with the prevention of chronic lung illnesses. The following are a few tips you can follow to prevent lung diseases.

Have a diet rich in fat, low in carbs

A reduction in carbs in your diet results in having a reduced production of carbon dioxide. This can help people who have lung disease in better management of health. A few studies have shown that people who followed the ketogenic diet had a low carbon dioxide output than people following the Mediterranean diet. When you reduce the carbs in your diet, make sure your healthy diet has many food choices.

Protein-rich foods

Eating high protein foods high in quality and grass-fed meat, fish, and poultry eggs is excellent. You need to make sure you eat food choices that include seafood, i.e., sardines and salmon.

Complex carbs

If you add carbs to your diet, choose complex carbs. These are the high foods in fiber, which helps them improve the digestive system's function and blood sugar management.

You can add the following foods to your diet:

- Peas
- Bran
- Lentils
- Beans
- Oats
- Barley
- Potatoes with skin

Fresh Produce

Fresh vegetables and fruits have all the essential minerals, vitamins, and fiber. These nutrients can help keep your body maintained and healthy. Non-starchy veggies, all without potatoes, peas, and corn, are less in carbs; hence they can add them to all diets. A few fruits and veggies are more stable than the rest.

Potassium-rich foods

Potassium is essential for proper lung function. Hence a potassium deficient may cause breathing issues. Try having the following foods that have higher levels of potassium, i.e.:

- Avocados

- Dark leafy greens

- Tomatoes

- Beets

- Asparagus

- Potatoes

- Bananas

- Oranges

Potassium-rich diets may be beneficial if the diet or the doctor has prescribed you the diuretic medication.

Healthy Fats

When choosing higher-fat diets, instead of choosing the fried foods, go for the meals and snacks that have fats such as nuts, avocadoes, coconut seeds and olives, olive fat, and cheese. These foods will give you more overall nutrition, mainly over the long run.

Stroke

What can you do to prevent having a stroke? Age makes us all a lot more susceptible to having issues like stroke. You cannot reverse the years or change the family history, but many such factors are linked to stroke that you may control, given that you are aware of them. Knowledge is a vast power. If you are aware of the particular risk factors that are sabotaging your health and are bringing your closer to other risk factors of stroke, you can take steps to eliminate the effects of this risk.

Choose the following food options for the prevention of stroke:

Eat many kinds of foods every day

Because no single food may provide our bodies with all the nutrients essential for our health, you must pick many kinds of foods to consume every day.

Eat many colorful foods for every meal

If you want to reap the most health-protective nutrients found in vegetables and fruits, it is essential to pick a rainbow of food colors for every meal. Pick the rainbow approach of choosing many kinds of fruits, legumes, and vegetables. You may have items that are dark red, deep green, vibrant yellow, purple and blue. By picking the whole rainbow color list, you will be surer to take a lot of nutrients.

Have or more cups of vegetables and fruits each day

Studies have shown that the best and ideal way to attain the most from your diet is to have as many fruits and vegetables as possible. In addition to the steps mentioned above, make sure you have 5 servings every day. A single serving that you have of vegetables should have:

- 1 cup of raw vegetables

- ½ cup of cooked vegetables

- 6 ounces vegetable juice

Read food labels

Reading the labels is just an ideal way to learn about the foods you are consuming. In law, most foods should have the nutritional information on their packaging's in the standard way. when you are picking the foods for dealing with risk factors of stroke, you should focus on the following information mainly:

- Calories

- Total fat

- Saturated fat

- Trans fat

- Cholesterol

- Sodium

- Dietary fiber

Alzheimer's

Alzheimer's disease is a very complex disorder for which doctors and specialists haven't devised any prevention or cure. But it is believed that the way we consume our food may be significantly linked to an increase or a decrease in the risk of Alzheimer's disease. Following are a few things you may do to prevent this disease at bay.

Eat many kinds of nutrients and low glycemic diet

Include such foods with vitamin C, E, and D in them and omega 3 fats and the antioxidants lutein and zeaxanthin. As it may happen with diabetes, researchers have suggested the production of higher levels of blood sugar and insulin may harm the brain and contribute to the progression of Alzheimer's.

Get regular exercise and also maintain an ideal weight

It will improve your immune system and blood pressure and act on your eye health and the brain. Being obese or overweight may increase your body's inflammation and boost the risk of developing many other diseases.

Keep the blood pressure and cholesterol regular

Having those cardiovascular diseases may contribute to the progression of having Alzheimer's disease.

Don't smoke

Toxins found in the first, second, and third-hand smoke may also be linked to the increase in having many diseases. Hence keeping away from it may help from honoring your memory for long.

Have a lot of good quality sleep

Having a good sleep quality keeps you active and present in your daily life routines and keeps you going strong with your mental health. Having a poor sleep may be significantly linked to developing a cognitive and memory issue.

Diabetes

Finding the best foods to have when you have diabetes may be a tough choice. It is because your primary goal must be to control blood sugar levels. It is also essential to eat foods that can help prevent diabetes complications such as heart diseases. The following diet options may be suitable for controlling diabetes.

Fatty Fish

Some people think fatty fish is the best and healthiest food on the plate. Salmon, herring, sardines, mackerel, and anchovies are the best sources for having omega 3 fatty acids EPA and DHA with many heart health benefits. Having enough of these fats continually is very important for people who have diabetes. EPA and DHA can protect the cells which line the blood vessels, reduce the markers of inflammation, and can also help to improve the function of your arteries.

Leafy Greens

Leafy greens are highly nutritious and are low in calories. They are also very low in digestible carbs or the carbs absorbed in the body, so they don't highly affect blood sugar levels. Kale, spinach, and many other leafy greens are a significant source of most vitamins and minerals, including **"Vitamin C"** having vitamin C can act like a potent antioxidant that shoes anti-inflammatory qualities as well.

Avocados

Avocados contain less than a gram of sugar, very few carbs, high fiber content, and healthy fats so that you don't have to worry about these items raising the blood sugar levels. Having avocado is linked to improved overall diet quality and a significant decrease in body weight and BMI. Avocado makes them just an ideal snack for people who have diabetes significantly as obesity may increase your chances of having diabetes.

Eggs

Eggs have many health benefits. They are those foods that can keep you feeling full for long in your meals. Constant egg consumption can help in the reduction of heart disease risks in many ways. Eggs reduce inflammation, increase the good HDL, improve insulin sensitivity, and modify the size and shape of the LDL cholesterol you have. Eggs are also an excellent source of lutein and antioxidants that may give you protection against most eye diseases.

Chia Seeds

Chia seeds are just a fantastic food choice for people who have diabetes. They're highly rich in fiber and are low in digestible carbs. They can also help in lowering your blood sugar levels. They can also slow down the speed at which your food moves in the gut and is absorbed.

Kidney Disease

You may protect the kidneys by managing the health conditions that can cause kidney damage. The steps that are given below can help you keep your kidneys healthy.

- Cook with a mixture of spices instead of just using salt

- Pick the veggies topics that include broccoli, spinach, and peppers.

- Try baking or just broiling the chicken, meat, and fish instead of just frying.

- Try to pick foods that have only a little or no added sugar.

- Eat foods made of whole grains include brown rice, whole wheat, whole grain, and oats.

- Slow the snack time down. Having a bag of that low-fat popcorn will take longer to eat than having a slice of cake.

- Try having a written record of all that you have been eating in a week. This may help you with keeping track of when you were overeating.

- Read the food labels. Pick the foods that have low saturated, trans fats, and cholesterol.

- Gradually move your way from whole milk to 2 percent of milk until you drink and cook in only fat-free or low-fat milk options.

These were a few ways you can keep your kidneys healthy. Your diet and nutrition play a huge role in maintaining your health and regulating your body systems. There are many ways you can make your diet better and improve your lifestyle to stay away from chronic diseases. You may also develop a strong fondness for healthy food options. Most people develop these habits of eating healthy, and hence they go a long way in their lives of staying young and active. You may also enjoy sound health in later years of life and have the same energy and health levels as when you were young.

Having a healthy diet is the best thing you can do for your body and also being active in daily life is a great option. Most people like having their predefined ways of enjoying their food choices. You may again do the same and win an active lifestyle in your later and more senior years.

Part 5

COOKING HEALTHY & NUTRITIOUS FOOD

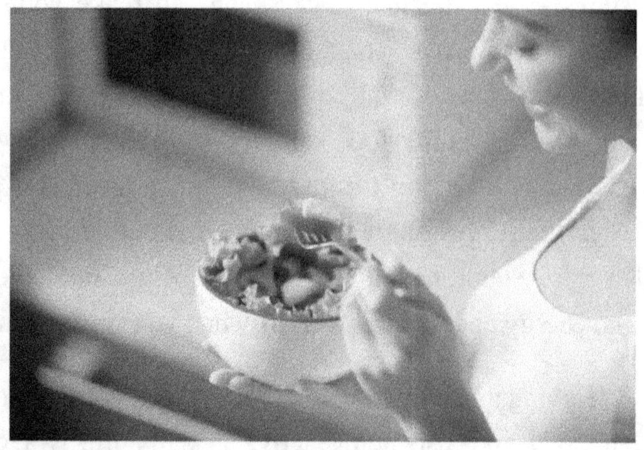

We may often be eating good food and think it to be healthy for our well-being, but the results are the opposite. This is because you may not be cooking your food the right way. There are a few ways you can harm your food's nutritional value as you are not cooking it well. A few ways to cook and process your meal perfectly to retain its nutritional value are given below.

1. Different Methods of Cooking

2. How cooking changes food

3. Preserving and keeping the essentials Nutrients in Cooked Food

Different Methods Of Cooking

The various methods of cooking your foods may impact the nutritional value of your foods significantly. You may obtain the maximum benefits of your food items if you cook them in ways that are identified as healthy cooking ways. Your favorite recipes may adapt quickly to give a healthy alternative. Take, for instance, nonstick cookware that may use to reduce the need for cooking oil. Vegetables may also be steamed or microwaved instead of only boiling them up to keep them full of nutrition. There are several ways to make your foods healthy. Limit the fats, salt, and sugars and add many fruits, vegetables, grains, low-fat dairy, and lawn meats in cooking. Foods that have added sugars, fats, or salts are a lot less healthy than foods that are found naturally.

Keep fats to a minimum

Select lean meats and reduced-fat dairy products and also limit the processed foods to only a minimum. Nuts, fish, seeds, soy, avocado, and olives are all healthy options as they have the essential long-chain fatty acids, and other good nutrients also accompany these fats. If you always add fats to your cooking, make sure you only keep them to a minimum and use monosaturated oils such as canola oil and olive oil.

Shop only healthy foods

Low-fat cooking starts when you are shopping for the items:

- Choose reduced or if it's a convenient low-fat conversion of the foods. You may take milk, yogurt, cheese, gravies, and salad dressings

- Choose lean meats and skinless chicken breasts

- Limit the chips, fast foods, crisps, pastries and pies, and processed meats with a considerable amount of fats in them.

Low-fat Cooking

A few suggestions for low-fat cooking are:

- If you have to use oil, try cooking sprays or apply only a small amount of oil using a pastry brush.

-   Cook in liquids such as wine, stock, fruit juice, lemon juice, vinegar, or water instead of oil.

-   Use low-fat yogurt, cornstarch, or evaporated skim milk instead of only using sauces or soups in cream.

-   When you are browning the vegetables, put them all in the hot pan and then spray on the oil instead of adding the oil first into the pan. Low-fat cooking will reduce the amount of oil that the vegetables will absorb while cooking.

-   The alternative to browning veggies using a pan-frying is to cook them in the microwave and then crisp them under a grill for a minute or two.

-   Use salsas, pesto, kinds of vinegar, and chutneys in the place of butter, sour creams, and creamy sauces.

Retaining the Nutrients

Water-soluble vitamins are exceptionally delicate, and they can quickly destroy while you are preparing food or cooking it. to minimize the loss, you may do the following:

- Scrub the vegetables instead of only peeling them, as most of the nutrients are present near the skin.

- Microwave or even steam the vegetables instead of only boiling them.

- If you prefer to cook the vegetables, utilize a small amount of water and make sure you do not overcook them.

- If you like boiling the vegetables, use a small portion of water and make sure you do not over boil them.

- Include a dry stir recipe in the diet. Stir-fried vegetable items are cooked a lot more quickly to have the crunch stored in them.

Cutting down the salt

Salt is a very common flavor booster, but research suggests that a high salt diet may contribute to many health issues, including high B.P. Suggestions on how you can reduce salt are as follows:

- Do not just randomly add salt to the food. Please make sure you taste it first.

- Add a splash of vinegar, olive oil, or lemon juice near the cooking end time or the cooked veggies. It may enhance the flavors just as the way salt does.

- Choose frozen or fresh vegetables as pickled or canned vegetables tend to be packed with salt.

- Limit the consumption of salty meat items such as ham, salami, bacon, corned beef, smoked salmon, chicken loaf, and frankfurters.

- Pick re reduced salt breakfast cereals and bread. Bread and cereals are also significant sources of salt in our diets.

Herbs

Culinary herbs are the plants that have leaves mainly and are used to add flavor and color in all kinds of meals. They are also active in giving your health-protective Phytoestrogens. In most cases, herbs can even replace the taste of oil and salt.

- Herbs are always very delicately flavored; hence add them to your cooking at the last minutes of cooking.

- Dried herbs are very strongly flavored than fresh ones. one teaspoon of the dried herbs is equal to four teaspoons of the fresh ones

- Apart from boosting the meat dishes, herbs may also add to bread, soups, slat dressings, mustards, desserts, drinks, and vinegar

- Herbs that include ginger, coriander, chili, garlic, and lemongrass are mainly complimentary in the vegetable-based recipes of stir fry

A Few General Suggestions

- Steam, grill, bake, boil, braise or microwave the foods

- Modify or eliminate the recipes that have butter in them or ask you to sauté or deep fry in the animal fat

- Avoid any added oils and butter or use nonstick cookware instead

- Don't just add salt to your foods as it is in the cooking.

- Remove the chicken skin and also trim the fat from the meat

- Eat fresh legumes and vegetables more

- Eat more fish that is high in protein and low in fat, and also loaded with the essential omega 3 fatty acids

How Cooking Changes Food

Eating healthy and nutritious foods may improve your energy levels and overall health. Surprisingly the way you are cooking your food also dramatically impacts the amounts of nutrients it has.

The nutrient content is mainly altered in the process of cooking

Cooking Food improves digestion and also increases the absorption of most nutrients. A few examples include the protein in the cooked eggs that is 180% high in being digestible than raw eggs. However, a few cooking methods may reduce many vital nutrients. The following are a few nutrients that get reduced while you are cooking:

- Water-soluble vitamins: vitamin C and B-thiamine, riboflavin, niacin, pyridoxine, pantothenic acid, cobalamin, folic acid

- Fat-soluble vitamins: Vitamin A, D, E, K

- Minerals: Primarily potassium, sodium, magnesium, calcium

Boiling, poaching and simmering

Boiling, poaching, and simmering are a few similar methods added in water-based cooking. These techniques mainly differ due to water temperature:

- Poaching: Less than 180 degrees F

- Simmering: 185 to 200 degrees F

- Boiling: 212 degrees F

Vegetables are mostly a great source of vitamin C, but a massive amount of them are mostly lost when cooked in water only. Boiling lessens vitamin C content way more than any other cooking process. Spinach, broccoli, and lettuce can lose up to 50% of higher vitamin C levels when boiled. As vitamin C is water-soluble and is also sensitive to heat, it may leach out the vegetables when boiling water. B vitamins are also susceptible to heat. Up to 60% of niacin, thiamine, and many other B vitamins may get lost when meta is simmered, and the juice runs off. However, when this liquid containing fluids is consumed, 100% of the minerals and 70 to 90% of B vitamins get retained. While on the other hand, boiling the fish may preserve omega 3 fatty acid content significantly more than microwaving or frying.

Grilling and Broiling

Grilling and broiling are the methods of cooling only with dry heat. When you are grilling, the heat source is obtained from only below, and when broiling, it comes from above. Grilling is the most popular kind of cooking method because of the very great taste it gives to the food. However, over 40% of B vitamins and minerals might be lost while grilling or broiling while the nutrient-rich juice drips off the meat. There are also a few concerns of polycyclic aromatic hydrocarbons that potentially cause cancers that form while the meat is grilled and the fat drips over the hot surfaces. However, researchers have also found that 41 to 89 percent may decrease pAHs if the drippings are removed and smoke minimized.

Microwaving

Microwaving is a convenient and safe method of cooking. Short times of cooking and the reduced exposure to heat keeps the nutrients preserved in the microwaved food. A few studies have found that microwaving is an ideal method of retaining the antioxidant activity present in garlic and mushrooms. Meanwhile, around 20 to 30 percent of vitamin C in the green vegetables gets lost while microwaving it. That is less than many cooking methods.

Roasting and Baking

Roasting and baking mean cooking in an oven using dry heat. Although these terms are interchangeable, roasting is the type of cooking used for meat, while baking is for bakery items, i.e., bread, cake, muffins, and similar foods. Most of the vitamin losses are minimal with this method of cooking, which includes vitamin C. However, due to the long cooking times at higher temperatures, B vitamins in the meat that has roasted may decline by over 40%.

Sautéing and stir-frying

With these cooking methods, foods are cooked in a saucepan over moderate or even high heat using only small amounts of oil or butter. These techniques are similar, but in stir-frying, the food is stirred very often, the temperature is high, and the cooking times are shorter. In general, it is a healthy way to prepare foods. Cooking only for a short time and not using water keeps the food from losing B vitamins, and also, the addition of fat improved the absorption of antioxidants and plant compounds.

Another study has found that the beta carotene absorption is 6.5 times higher in the stir-fried carrots than in the raw ones. In another study, blood lycopene levels also increased by 80% when people have tomatoes sauteed in olive oil instead of any of it. Store frying has also been shown to reduce vitamin C amounts significantly in broccoli and red cabbage.

Frying

Frying involves cooking foods in high amounts of fat that is primarily oil on higher temperatures. The food is then coated with bread crumbs or batter. It is a popular way of preparing most food items as the skin, or the coatings maintain a seal that ensures that the insides remain the most and cook evenly. The fat that is used for the frying process makes the food very tasty. However, not all foods can be fried. Fatty fish is the ideal source of omega 3 fatty acids that have many health benefits.

But these fats are very delicate and are prone to damage at higher temperatures. Frying tuna has shown degradation in the omega 3 content up to 70 to 85%, whereas baking causes a slight loss. In contrast, the drying process preserves vitamin C and B vitamins and can also increase the amount of fiber in potatoes by converting the starch into resistant starch. When the oil is heated up to higher temperatures for an extended period, aldehydes are formed, toxic substances. Aldehydes have been linked to the increase of cancer risk and many other diseases.

Preserving And Keeping The Essentials Nutrients In Cooked Food

Having nutritious food to eat may improve your health and energy levels. The foods that we consume consist of fats, carbs, proteins, minerals, and vitamins. These are the substances that are known as nutrients. We need nutrients for the following:

- For energy to carry out our daily tasks

- To grow

- To repair our body

- To keep us protected from diseases and infections

The food we consume is rich in one or other nutrition, but none of the foods give us all of the essential nutrients. We require all of the nutrients to maintain energy, growth, and our healthy body. We must include all food items that are rich in various nutrients in our foods. We must consist of such foods that are rich in nutrients in our diets. Such a diet that has a balance of all the essential nutrients is known as a balanced diet.

Carbs

Carbohydrates are highly energy-giving foods. Carbohydrates are found in items that are:

- Dairy products that include yogurt, milk, and ice cream

- Fruits that have whole fruits and fruit juices

- Grains that include rice, bread, and cereal

- Vegetables that include potatoes and corns

- Sugars and the sweet food items

Fats

Fats give us high energy levels. Fats are needed but not in that excess. Excessive fats get stored in the body and clog our blood vessels resulting in many heart illnesses. Food items that provide us fats are cheese, nuts, chocolates, meat, whole eggs, oils, ghee, etc.

Proteins

Proteins are high bodybuilding foods. They help us in the repair of the growth of the body. They help in building muscles. We get proteins from fish, eggs, cheese, milk, and chicken.

Vitamins and Minerals

Vitamins and minerals keep us protected from falling ill. Vitamins and minerals keep us healthy. They are known as protective food. We get minerals and vitamins from fruits, milk, and vegetables. Minerals are needed for stronger teeth and bones. Milk is highly rich in minerals and vitamins such as calcium. Calcium keeps our bones and teeth strong. We must eat a lot of fruits while it's summer as fruits help our bodies stay hydrated. Vitamin C is essential for building immunity, and immunity helps us to fight against infections and viruses. Citrus fruits such as lemons and oranges are a rich source of vitamin C. water helps our digestion, and it also regulates our body temperature. The average adult human body is composed of 50 to 60 % of water. Roughage is the indigestible part of vegetables, grains, and fruits. It assists the process of digestion.

Food Preservation

Food preservation is the process of preserving our foods and keeping them fresh for a long time. there are many kinds and methods of food preservation that are as follows:

Drying

A few foods are fried to keep them preserved over a long period. Most people dry fruits and maintain them to use them out of season.

Freezing or Refrigeration

A few foods are frozen to keep the taste preserved and upkeep the nutritional value, such as peas being taken out of their pods and frozen.

Pickling

Pickling is one other famous type of preservation of food. Food items are fried in oil, such as mustard oil, and are kept for more extended periods.

Fermentation

Food preservation is famously done through the process of fermentation. Items are fermented and stored for more extended periods to give their best flavor, such as wines.

Canning

Vegetables and meat, and some other food items are preserved through canning. A syrup is left in them to keep the things full of nutritional value.

Sweetening

When sugar is added to the food items, it starts killing the germs. Sugar is also added to bring some taste to things such as jams and jelly.

Salting

Fishes and some such items are dehydrated by salting them. This process is used to keep these items consumable for more extended periods. These were a few ways of preserving food items so that they can consume in later months. This process of keeping food fresh for long and also for non-seasonal times is ancient. When people didn't have refrigerators, or they had only a few seasons when food was available, they used to preserve the food to keep it consumable over the year. Still, people use this process to bring the best taste out of the food items and keep them fresh. These processes of preserving food do not make food items lose their nutritional value. You may enjoy the health benefits of pickled foods and other preserved foods by having them at any time of the day.

When done right, we can permanently preserve the nutritional content of foods and do our best not to lose their nutritional value. Many people keep these items fresh for long and can keep them looking healthy without losing the flavor. You can enjoy these foods out of season and take their beneficial nutritional advantage that our bodies need throughout different seasons of the year.

Nutrients present in vegetables and fruits break down from when they were first harvested to the time they were ready to be consumed. This loss in nutrients may be minimized by a proper storage method or through prepping. You can protect the foods by keeping them away from higher temperatures. You can store them in cooler climates. Use dedicated food rotation labels to keep the FIFO maintained for storage and handling. Do not slice the vegetables too far ahead, and make sure you store them intact. Cut the product which needs to be cooked over long into more significant pieces, exposing the fewer surfaces from vitamins that can be lost.

So, are you ready to keep your foods preserved for long so that you don't have to wait for summers to enjoy those ripe mangoes or for winters to enjoy orange marmalade jam?

Part 6

THE AMOUNT OF NUTRITION YOU NEED

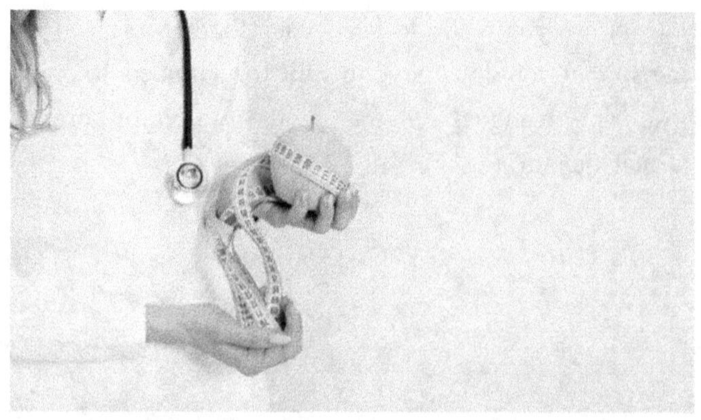

Knowing how much nutrition your body needs to keep performing correctly will help you maintain your health. You can keep your bodily functions working correctly even at old age if you take only as much food as needed. A guide to healthy nutrition may educate you about the importance of eating well.

1. DRI: Complete Guideline for Healthy Nutrition

2. RDAs: Prescription for Good Food

3. ALS: Food Safety and Quality

A balanced diet is vital for your body as it provides your body the nutrients that it needs to work correctly. To get this nutrition's you should consume the following items so that most of your calories are coming from them:

Fresh fruits

Fresh vegetables

Whole grains

Legumes

Nuts

Lean protein

Through the following three, you will get the most nutrition and build a strong body and learn about healthy foods for you. But let's find out other aspects of the nutrition that your body requires to function normally and let you enjoy a healthy life. Following is a detailed guide on the food that you need.

Dri: Complete Guideline For Healthy Nutrition

Since 1998, the Institute of Medicine has release 8 total volumes of DRIs, which offer quantitative estimates over the nutrient intakes to be used in the process for assessing and planning diets that apply to all healthy individuals in the U.S. and Canada.

These 8 volumes are then summarized in the Reference volume name Dietary Reference Intakes: The Essential Reference for Dietary Planning and Assessment. Organized by the nutrient for ready use, this reference volume reviews every nutrient's function in the human body, usual dietary intakes, food sources, and effects of excessive intakes and deficiencies.

DRI is the abbreviation for Dietary Reference Intakes. These are the documents issued by the Food and Nutrition Board of the Institute of Medicine, National Sciences Academy. The Board of Food and Nutrition addresses the issues regarding safety, adequacy, and quality of the food supply, builds the principles and guidelines of proper and adequate dietary intake, and renders authoritative judgments over the relationships among nutrition, food intake, and health.

DRI is a general term for the set of reference values planned and assess healthy people's nutrient intakes.

These values are varied depending on age and sex, which are stated below:

- Recommended Dietary Allowances (RDA): an average daily level of the consumption of sufficient items to meet the nutrient requirements of almost all healthy people.

- Adequate Intake (A.I.): it is established when the evidence is insufficient to form an RDA and is mostly set at the level assumed to ensure the adequacy of nutrients.

- Tolerable Upper Intake Level (U.L.): the maximum and a daily intake to give adverse health outcomes.

The DRI is a set of reference rules used to plan and assess all healthy people's nutrient intakes. They are used widely for:

- Designing and then evaluating research studies and their results

- Developing the dietary guidelines and food guides

- Planning and keeping track of nutrition-related public health programs and dietary intakes for military personnel

- Creating consumer and patient counseling and all educational programs

The U.S. and Canadian governments have formed a Federal DRI committee that works together to recognize DRI needs and coordinate governed sponsorships of the DRI reviews and their activities.

The U.S. and Canadian Governments have also jointly funded a 2019 report on the DRIs for potassium and sodium. As they follow this, the National Academies of Sciences, Engineering, and Medicine (NASEM) has formed an educational webpage known as the Expansion of the dietary Reference intake Model: Learning from Sodium and Potassium.

The Guiding Principles For Chronic Disease Endpoints And DRIs:

The Joint U.S. Canadian DRI Working Group has sponsored a National Academies of Sciences, Engineering, and Medicine (NASEM) consensus study during the summer of 2016. This study was designed to inform about the principles that committees can use to include the chronic disease endpoints when setting future DRIs. DRIs built the project on the workshop of March 2015, panel discussion, and this workshop's report. The NASEM report's guiding principles for Developing

Dietary Reference Intakes Based on Chronic Disease were finished and released in August 2017.

Dietary Reference Intakes and chronic Disease Endpoint Workshop and Report: The March 2015 Dietary Reference Intakes and Chronic Disease Endpoints Workshop and the lengthy and descriptive follow-up discussions informed the report's development basing Dietary Reference Intakes (DRIs) on the chronic disease endpoints.

RDAs: Prescription For Good Food

The RDA that is the estimation of Recommended Dietary Allowance is the estimated amount of nutrition or calories per day are considered necessary for the maintenance of excellent health by the Food and Nutrition Board of National Research Council and National Academy of Sciences. The RDA is updated in periods to reflect the newly obtained knowledge. It is correctly known as the Recommended Daily Allowance.

RDA is the minimum daily intake that fulfills almost all of the healthy people in a very particular life stage or a group. It is the average daily dietary intake level that gets sufficient to meet the nutritional requirements of almost all healthy people of a particular sex, age, physiological condition, or life stage. The RDA is the nutrient intake goal to plan the diets of people.

To ensure that these needs of any given person are met, a variability measure around eth EAR, using the standard deviation and otherwise if data is insufficient, an estimated coefficient of variation of 10 to 15% is assumed. Then the amount which covers this variation is assessed. The RDA is hence defined through two standard deviations above EAR, assuming a normal distribution of nutrient requirements as it can be for most of the nutrients that are studied. That is, RDA is the EAR + 2 S.D. If this standard deviation is not available, using the CV of 10%, RDA is set at 1.2 times the EAR. If the CV is assumed to be 15%, the RDA is then placed at 1.3 times the EAR.

The rich, but not a certainty of inadequacy, then increases as the intakes fall below the RDA. However, the RDA is the overly generous criterion for evaluating nutrient adequacy. By definition, RDA exceeds the actual requirements of all but around 2 to 3% of the whole population. Hence, many individuals below RDA might still have enough of the nutrient that is in question to be over their requirement level.

The 1989 RDA has a single reference point that focuses on achieving sufficient only for the individuals. However, the reference was mostly mistaken and was applied as the standard for evaluating population nutrient intakes. RDA is not the appropriate tool for assessing individuals' diets or assessing the planning of group diets.

ALS: Food Safety And Quality

ALS gives you an unrivaled choice of drinks and food testing services for an extensive range of food choices. ALS has highly experienced food experts of the industry that can help with the eth food safety and quality program you are running. Having a suite of many testing services at hand, ALS can assist in food safety management in diverse industries to ensure product compliance is achieved.

Is there anyone who may say that food isn't that important to our lives? Moreover, at first, food is our fuel. Therefore, with all certainly, they are essential for our existence. Hence food being all that helps us function and move around in a way that allows us to exist should have quality. The food which enters the house must be in its ideal condition. Like any vehicle would need quality fuel so that it won't erode or spoil, it does with us. Hence, food quality and safety tests are unnecessary and highly essential to provide the ideal consumption.

The importance of analysis of food

Food safety is essential. Not only for people who manufacture it but also for those who consume it. Once an exact composition of food is achieved, it becomes wholly possible to warn about all of the precautions and the rest of the protection. In short, the process is routine quality control. While the food components are being evaluated, the state of the raw materials is also done. It is the characteristics that control the processing of foods. In other words, the analysis for food safety is critical not only to ensure quality but also for thorough care and inspection.

What is Analyzed

Food safety through the process of food analysis recognizes many various aspects of food. But it ranges from the chemical composition, the interaction it has with the human body, and the packaging. Below you may see what is analyzed.

- Chemical composition

- Action in the organism

- Food and its caloric value

- Physical properties

- Chemical properties

- Physiological properties

- Possible adulterants and contaminations

The types of food analysis

The safety of food is essential, but it also exists in many kinds with many varied functions. After all, your food is highly rich in possibilities and hence presents many paths of analysis. It is explained below:

Microscopic analysis

In short, the goal behind it is to find foreign materials for products. Microscopic examination is not natural to it and is not visible to our naked eye, and plastics, stones, and some like it.

Microbiological analysis

Equally effective to acquire food safety. This analysis keeps an eye on the microorganisms that may cause harm to people who consume them. Elements that are detrimental to our human bodies are what this analysis finds out. Through this analysis, this company not only keeps the public protected but also protects the products. This way, it is recognized as safer for the food to be commercialized in the market. Besides, it may be required by law; hence it is only performed in the accredited labs.

Sensory analysis

As a result of the organic research, it comes with the sole purpose of investigating all of the sensory aspects. It serves to find out the smell, visual reactions to taste and touch, and its sounds. It is also worth noting that this analysis may analyze the final products, the raw materials, and the intermediate production stages.

Physical analysis in food

Do you know about the nutritional table of the foods you eat? Then much of that information is then collected in the physical-chemical research. As the food safety guidelines suggest, this analysis helps in quality control and elaborates the label.

DNA Test

How can it be possible that the consumer having food knows with an absolute surety that the food is his nature? In a few other words, take, for example, is beef? That is why there is DNA testing. It is carried out along with eth purpose of ensuring that products of animals and vegetables origin are of the species purchase. The DNA test is essential to food safety. You may know a lot more about food safety tests.

ALS is designed to help meet the environment's regulatory needs. They offer customers accurate, legally defensible, and analytical data, giving the customers an extensive range of accredited analytical services for land, water, and waste monitoring. ALS environment is the biggest U.K.'s leading provider in analytical services.

Through working with the customers for over twenty years, they at ALS have developed a range of many analytical services that meet the specific needs, including the standard industry, bespoke analytical, and regulatory suites.

They can also respond in a timely and efficient manner to the sampling and analytical needs through the network of service centers and labs in the U.K. and Ireland.

Part 7

FIVE AUTHENTIC NUTRITION WEBSITES

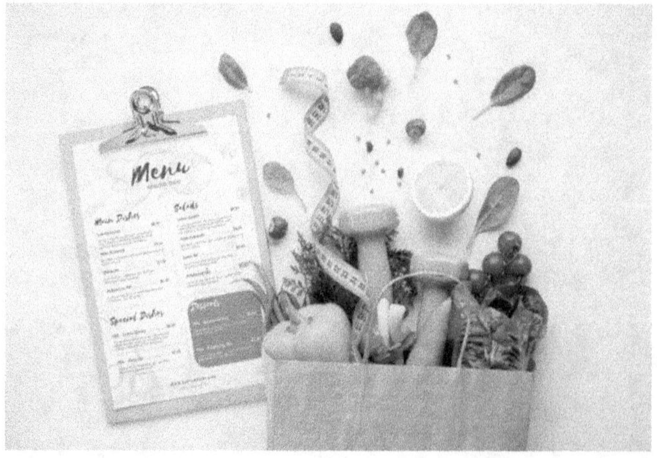

You don't need to trust vague and non-authentic sources on nutrition and its effect on the body when we have handpicked the following most authentic sources. Our information is based on these sources, and they are trusted by people worldwide in means of being a credible source of information.

1. **U.S. Department of Agriculture (USDA) Nutrient Database**

2. **U.S. Food and Drug Administration (FDA)**

3. **Academy of Nutrition and Dietetics (AND)**

4. **Food Allergy Research & Education (FARE)**

5. **American Cancer Society**

U.S. Department Of Agriculture (USDA) Nutrient Database

Food Data Central is the integrated data system that provides expanded nutrient profile data and links to related agriculture and experimental research. At this moment, only a basic view of the search results is available for seeing on mobile devices. Advanced filter features, including searching by data type, do not enable mobile yet and are only viewable on desktop. Users are now encouraged to use the desktop computer to carry out food item searches.

Food Data Central takes the analysis, presentation, and compilation of nutrient and food component data to a higher level.

Food Data Central

- May be used by and has benefits for many users, including policymakers, researchers, academicians and educators, nutrition and health professionals, product developers, etc.

- Includes five distinct and different data types which provide the information on food and profiles of nutrients: Foundation Foods, Food and Nutrient Database for the dietary studies 2017-2018 (FNDDS 2017 – 2018), National Nutrient Database for the Standard Reference Legacy Release (S.R. Legacy), Experimental Foods and USDA Global Branded Food Producer Database. Each of these is the data type that has a unique purpose and also unique attributes.

- Links these distinct data types into one location, strengthening policymakers, researchers, and others to address all the vital issues related to food, diet health interactions, and nutrition.

- Gives a broad snapshot within the time of the nutrients and other components found in a large variety of foods and food products.

- The Food supply and scientific understanding of various dietary intakes and healthy relationships have been evolving. USDA's food composition data resources are also changing to meet the requirements of diverse users. In the past few years, the fastly escalating pace of the change in food supply and a growing variety of food data uses have massively enhanced the requirement for transparent and piece of easily accessible information on the nutrients and many other components in food and food products. This need requires a whole new approach to analyzing, compiling, and presenting food profile information in the scientifically rigorous method. Food Data Central continues to embody the new system.

- Food Data Central contains the five distinct types of data that give information on the nutrients and other food components. However, these data types have unique purposes and attributes and can be used in eth complementary ways to acquire various research and related objectives. The two data types are Foundation Foods and Experimental Foods. They provide data that have never been previously available. These data types will focus on efforts as Food Data Central is expanded and developed in the coming years.

- Foundation Foods are the ones that include values for nutrients and all other food components in a very diverse range of foods and the ingredients and also the underlying metadata. These metadata include the sample numbers, sampling location, analytical approaches used, date of collection, and, if appropriate, the agricultural information, including genotype and production practices. The enhanced depth and transparency of Foundation Foods data may provide valuable insights into the many factors influencing food and nutrient component profiles' variability.

- Experimental foods have foods produced, acquired, and studied under many unique conditions such as alternative management systems, experimental genotypes, and analytical protocols. The foods in this kind of data may not be available commercially to the general public; data may also expand information on the specific food. Experimental foods are only for research purposes and may not be referred to the consumer for the diet planning data of Experimental Foods.

U.S. Food And Drug Administration (FDA)

The FDA is responsible for keeping public health protected by ensuring the efficacy, safety, and security of human and veterinary drugs, biological products, and medical devices and ensuring the safety of the nation's food supply, products, and cosmetics emit radiation. The FDA also has the responsibility to regulate the manufacturing, distribution, and marketing of tobacco products to produce public health and reduce tobacco use by minors.

FDA is also responsible for the advancements of public health through helping to speed up the innovations that make medical products a lot more effective, safe and affordable and helping the public get accurate, science-based information. They need to utilize the medical products and also the foods to maintain and even improve their health.

FDA also plays a vital role in the Nations' terrorism capability. The FDA fulfills the responsibility by ensuring the security of the food supply and fostering medical products' development to respond to the deliberate and naturally emerging public health threats.

FDA's Regulatory Responsibilities: Laws and Regulations:

- Laws enforced by FDA

- What does FDA help regulate

- FDA 101: An overview of the FDA's regulatory and the research activities

- FDA regulations: 21 CFR, Drugs and Food

Product Approval

- Approvals of FDA regulated products

- Is it really "FDA approved?"

Recalls, News, and Events:

- Recalls, safety alerts, and market withdrawals

- FDA news and events

Guidance documents, Freedom of information, and rulemaking

- Search for the FDA guidance documents

- FDA rules and regulations

- FDA Dockets: Comment on Administrative proceedings and rulemaking

- Freedom of Information

FDA is the agency in the Department of Health and Human Services. Effective from 31st march, 2019, FDA started the operational implementation of the agency reorganization. FDA's reorientation always reflects the agency's commitment to modernizing its structure to start advancing its mission to protect and promote public health and meet the challenges of rapid innovation across the industries regulated through the FDA. The FDA's reorganization will also realign many agency entities to promote many strategic priorities and elevate centers, field forces, and offices.

FDA is the most senior comprehensive consumer protection agency working in the U.S. federal government. Since 1848 the federal government has been using eth chemical analysis to monitor many agriculture products' safety, a responsibility inherited by the Department of Agriculture in 1862 and later by the FDA. Although it wants to be known by the present name until1 930, FDA had its modern regulatory functions started with the passage of the 1906 Pure Food and Drugs Act, which is law a quarter-century in the making which prohibited interstate commerce in misbranded and adulterated food and drugs.

These had been eth driving force behind the law and headed its enforcement over eth early years, giving essential protection elements that the consumers didn't even know before that time. Since then, the FDA has also changed along with economic, social, political, and legal changes in the U.S. The history of these changes illuminates the ever-evolving role. The FDA has played in promoting public health and offers lessons to consider as we evaluate current regulatory challenges.

Academy Of Nutrition And Dietetics (AND)

The Academy of Nutrition and Dietetics is the world's most prominent organization of food and nutrition professionals founded in Cleveland, Ohio, in 1917 by a group of visionary women dedicated to helping the government conserve food and improve the health of the public in World War I. Today this academy stands for over 100,000 credential practitioners, registered dietitian nutrition, wrote dietetic technicians, and other dietetics and nutrition professionals holding undergraduate and advanced degrees in dietetics and nutrition and students. It is devoted to improving the nation's health and advancing the dietetics profession using research, education, and advocacy.

Members of this academy play a key role in shaping the public's food choices, improving the nutritional status, and treating people with injuries and illnesses. Members offer several preventative and medical nutrition therapy services in many settings. Nutrition and dietetics experts work in health care systems, food service, home health care, research, business and education organizations, and public spaces. As the vital members of medical teams in hospitals and the long-term care facilities and health maintenance organizations, they offer medical nutrition therapy through specific nutrition services to deal with chronic conditions, injuries, and illnesses.

Community-based dietetics practitioners are working to provide health promotion, wellness services, and disease prevention. As a nutrition and food issue leader, the academy offers expert testimony on hearings, lobbies Congress and the other governmental bodies, develops position statements on critical nutrition and food issues, and comments on proposed federal and state regulations.

The vision of the academy of nutrition and dietetics is to achieve a world where all people thrive through a transformative power of nutrition and food. The mission is to accelerate the improvements in global health and well-being using food and nutrition. These principles include:

- Amplify the contribution of dietetics and nutrition practitioners and also expand the workforce capacity and capability

- Integrate the research, technology, professional development, and practice to stimulate the innovation and discovery

- Collaborate for solving the most excellent food and nutrition challenges that are being faced now and also in eth future e

- Focus on the system-wide impact across many foods, health care sectors, and well being

- Has a global effect on eth elimination of all forms of malnutrition.

Foundation Initiatives

The only charitable organization dedicated solely to nutrition and dietetics is the Academy of Nutrition and Dietetics Foundation. Their vision is we all eat right. Focusing on the four key initiatives, scholarship, food, awards, and nutrition research, and public education related to the kids. Eat right and the future of food. This foundation I dedicated to advancing public health and nutrition are utilizing the expertise of registered dietician nutritionists.

Future of Food

The Future of Food initiative's initial work is to engage nutrition and hunger relief professionals to increase food insecurity awareness while promoting access to healthy foods and quality nutrition education in the food banks.

Kids Eat Right

The Academy of Nutrition and Dietetics and the Academy of Nutrition and Dietetics and Foundation launched their first joint initiative, Kids Eat Right, in November 2010. This member-driven campaign is highly dedicated to supporting the whole house's efforts to end the childhood obesity epidemic in the generation.

Food Allergy Research & Education (FARE)

FARE enhances people's lives with food allergies empowering them to live a safe and productive life with respect from other people. FARE's efforts in eth research, education, advocacy, and awareness support people with food allergies to live productive and safe lives with others' respect. The 2020 impact Report outlines the Fares' incredible accomplishments over the past 12 months and spotlights not only the existing program growth and organization influence but also puts light on the exciting new projects that are currently taking shape and are being positioned to real the impact in 2021 and beyond.

FARE has been highly dedicated to expanding beyond traditional vehicles of line. They have launched the Living Teal brand to build and embrace the broader food allergy community, with an engaging and fun lifestyle content designed to share tips, heartwarming stories, and recipes on how we may all live the best lives by Living Teal. These platforms let them offer the community while presenting information in new and entertaining formats and also emphasizing what is most important in a more engaging way than is possible through the status quo.

FARE is also committed to reversing the rising prevalence of food allergies. New research led by FARE's chief medical officer for the Public Health, MPH, shows that only 30 percent of U.S. pediatricians are ultimately sharing the early peanut introduction guide to the new parents. No guidance has ever been developed to stop the rise of the remaining top allergies of food. It is taking action to boost the awareness of the benefits of early introduction to food allergy prevention initiatives. This transformational program aims to reduce the growth of a potentially life-threatening food allergy among infants and young kids and slow the rise of food allergies overall.

SEED: exploring Early introduction to inform physicians better, government and parents

It is grounded in the success of the 2015 Learning Early About Peanut Allergy (LEAP_ study and bolstered through the support of any top-caliber partners, FARE has launched the Start Eating Early Diet (SEED) program. Alongside Northwestern University Feinberg School of Medicine, Ann and Robert H. Lurie Children's Hospital of Chicago, the SEED study will find out the potential benefits of the early introduction of multiple allergenic foods, specifically peanut, dairy, egg, soy, cashew, almond, and sesame in a very radical, racial and socioeconomic sample of infants.

How SEED will change Food allergy:

To address the challenges limited in previous studies, Phase One of the SEE study kicked off during November 2020 with the national survey to assess attitudes, needs, and barriers to introducing allergenic foods. Age-appropriate foods and recipes will give infant caregivers assurance that cost and access do not limit participation. In addition to this, the babies at average risk of food allergy, high-risk infants will be listed in the precise evaluation of the effectiveness of systemic feeding of multiple allergenic foods for allergy prevention.

FARE is working with the food manufacturers and food allergy advocacy organizations to develop the new standardized and voluntary food allergen precautionary labeling system and support the new label with the information. Educational campaigns geared to individuals and families from diverse socioeconomic backgrounds help consumers make informed decisions when they shop. FARE has held over 50 briefings and has also communicated the impactful study's findings to over 200 food manufacturers, government agencies, and associations.

American Cancer Society

The American Cancer Society is a nationwide, community-based voluntary health organization dedicated to eliminating cancer as the primary health issue. There Global Headquarters are located in Georgia, Atlanta, and they also have regional and local offices in the country to make sure they have a presence in every community. Their mission is to see how the local and international American Cancer Society strives to live with a clearly defined set of goals and ideals. These core values are used as a light to guide the way through decision-making and planning. We learn how to save lives every day as we work to form a world free from pain and suffering from cancer.

The American Cancer Society was found in 1913 by 10 doctors and 5 other laypeople in New York City. It was known as the American Society for the Control of Cancer (ASCC). During that time, the cancer diagnosis meant only near-certain death. Rarely ever mentioned in public, the disease was steeped in denial and fear. A few times, doctors did not also tell their patients they have cancers, and the patients also didn't tell their family and friends that they have been diagnosed.

The society has founders who knew they needed to raise public awareness of cancer if the American cancer society made progress against the disease. Despite the enormity of the task, the founders of the American Cancer Society and the colleagues set about writing articles for Popular magazines and many professional journals, publishing the campaign Notes a monthly bulleting of cancer information, and the recruitment of doctors throughout the country to help in the education of the public.

During those years, the society first used its iconic Sword of Hope symbol that today is part of its logo. This sword came from the 1928 nationwide poster contest by ASCC.

The American Cancer Society invests hundreds of millions of dollars each year to globally fight off cancer and has earned public trust by demonstrating a history of careful and proven financial stewardship for more than a century. They raised nearly all of the money through private individual donations that help to make sure their independence. They encourage people to look at how effectively they deliver their mission and how efficiently they are operating. We are also deeply committed to the reporting of shareholders, i.e., the millions of people that support them every year.

American Cancer Society is committed to eth efficiency and transparency. Also, it relies on direct mail and special events, including Relay for Life, Determination, Making Strides Against Breast Cancer,

CEOs Against Cancer for the maintenance of their vital volunteers. The donor base and the public's education and information regarding cancer prevention, its early detection, and patient programs are offered and are available for them. The society also utilizes the events to drive the call to action for cancer prevention and the screenings and public policy advocacy.

This educational and information delivery is directly inherent in their mission statement to save, celebrate lives, and lead the fight for a world free of cancer. They communicate and educate the postal mail, telephone, digitally, and in person at the events not to generate income only but to fulfill our mission. As a result, by the Financial Accounting Standards Board (FASB) guidance and the Internal Revenue Service (IRS) guidelines, they allocate a portion of their direct mail and the special event costs to program services.

As a nonprofit organization exempt from any federal taxation, we ensure donors' money is spent as ideally and effectively as possible.

Part 8

SELF ASSESSMENT CHART

As long as you cannot assess yourself the right way daily, you aren't doing fine. You need to know your progress level and must be able to determine if the natural diets are helping you achieve your ideal figure or not. The following chart will help you gain an insight into how much you ate today and the nutritional value you are consuming daily.

Every five years, the Department of Health and Human Services and the Department of Agriculture issue a report which contains the nutritional and dietary information and the guidelines for the general public over the past two years of age based on the review of scientific-based evidence. The aim is to advise promoting health and reducing the risk for major chronic illnesses through diet and physical activity. A detailed description of the process and also the most recent report is also included in many posts.

From this website of Health Government, you may find the following:

- Balance the calories through physical activity to manage weight

- Consume high levels of certain foods and nutrients that include vegetables, fruits, fat-free, whole grains and low-fat dairy products, and also seafood

- Consume lesser foods with sodium, i.e., salt, trans fats, saturated fats, added sugars, cholesterol, and refined grains.

The Dietary Guidelines for Americans, 2010 includes 23 key recommendations for a general population and six additional vital recommendations for specific population groups such as pregnant women. The recommendations are intended so that people that choose an overall healthy diet can be helped.

Major Recommendations

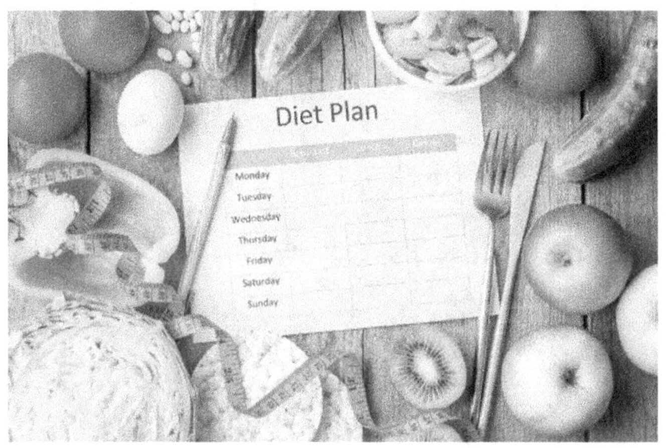

Manage weight

- Prevent and also reduce overweight and obese people through improved eating and even physical activity behaviors

- Control total calorie intake for the management of body weight. For people that are overweight or are obese, this will mean having lesser calories from beverages and foods

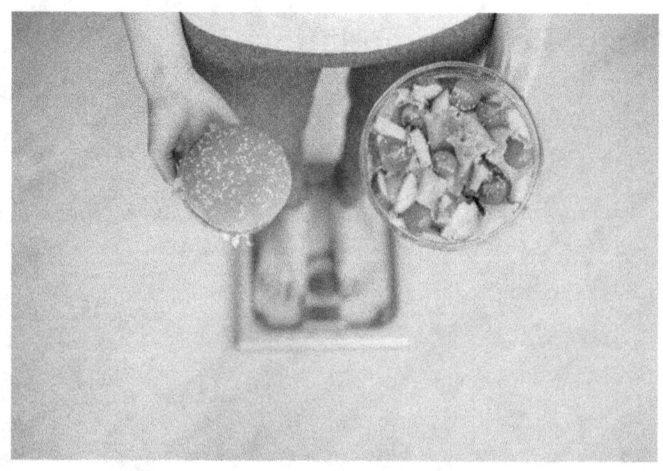

- Increase physical activity and also reduce the time spent in sedentary behaviors

- Maintain the appropriate calorie balance in each stage of life, childhood, adulthood, adolescence, breastfeeding, and pregnancy, and old age people.

Foods and food components to reduce

Reduce a daily sodium intake to fewer than 2,300 milligrams and further reduce the information to 1,500 mg among 51 and older people and those of any age who are African American or have diabetes, hypertension, or chronic kidney illness. - The 1,500 mg recommendation applies to almost half of the U.S. population, which includes children as well and a majority of adults

- Consume lesser than 10 percent of calories from the saturated fatty acids through the replacement of them with monosaturated and polyunsaturated fatty acids

- Consume less than 300 mg/ per of dietary cholesterol

- Keep trans fatty acid consumption as little as possible by the limitation of foods that have synthetic sources of trans fats that include partially hydrogenated oils and also by limited other solid fats

- Reduction of the intake of calories from added sugars and solid fats

- Limit the consumption of such foods that have refined grains, especially the refined grain foods which have solid fats, sodium, and added sugars

- If alcohol is consumed, it must be taken in moderate amounts up to only a drink per day for women and only two drinks per day for men and only by adults if they are of legal drinking age

Foods and Nutrients to increase

- Individuals must meet the following suggestions as a part of a healthy eating pattern while they are staying in the calorie needs

- Increase the intake of vegetables and fruits

- Eat a whole variety of vegetables, especially dark greens, oranges, red vegetables, and peas and beans.

- Consume almost half of all of the grains as whole grains. Increase the intake of whole grains by the replacement of refined grains with the whole grains

- Increase an intake of fat-free or low-fat milk products, which include yogurt, milk, cheese, or the fortified soy beverage

- Choose the variety of protein foods that include seafood, poultry, lean meat, beans, eggs, unsalted nuts and seed, and soy products

- Increase the amount and the kinds of seafood consumed by selecting types of seafood in the place of meat and poultry.

- Replace the protein foods that are abundant with the solid fats with choices that are lower in solid fats and calories or the sources of oils

- Use oils for the replacement of solid fat wherever possible

- Choose the foods which provide higher potassium, calcium, dietary fiber, vitamin D that are the nutrients of concern in most American diets. These foods are fruits, vegetables, whole grains, and milk, and their products

Recommendations For Specific Population Groups

Women capable of being Pregnant

- Pick the foods which supply heme iron that is more readily absorbed by our bodies, additional sources of iron, and enhancers of iron absorption that is vitamin C rich foods

- Consume 400 mcg/day of synthetic folic acid in addition to food forms of the folate from a varied kind of diet

- Women who are pregnant or are breastfeeding

- Consume 8 to 12 ounces of foods from the sea that is more readily absorbed in the body, additional iron sources, and the enhancers of iron absorption, which includes vitamin C rich foods

- Due to the higher amount of methyl mercury in white tuna, it should be limited to only 6 ounces per week and should not be eaten if it is from these four types, i.e., shark, tilefish, swordfish, and king mackerel

- If pregnant, take the iron supplements recommended by the obstetrician or the other health care provider.

Individual at ages 50 years or more

- Consume foods that are fortified with vitamin B12, which includes cereals or dietary supplements.

Building healthy eating Patterns

- Select the eating pattern which meets all of the nutrition needs overtime at an appropriate calorie level intake

- Account for all of the foods and beverages that are consumed and assess how they fit in a total healthy eating pattern

- Follow the food safety recommendations when preparing and eating foods to reduce the risk of foodborne disease.

Dietary Self-Assessment

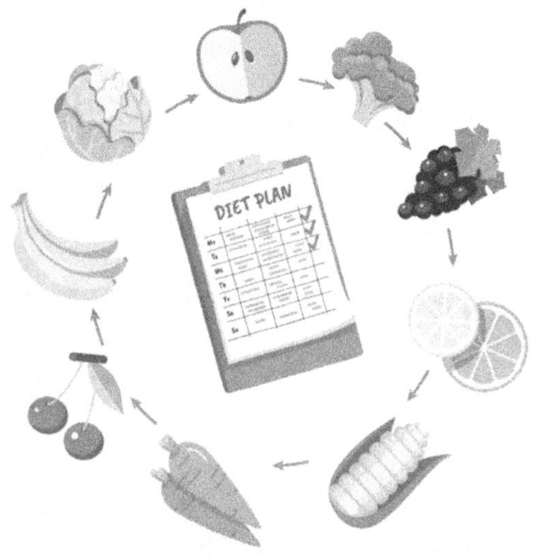

The dietary self-assessment must have the following four essential elements:

Pre-assessment Reflection

Before starting the self-assessment, you must ask yourself how you receive health based on the weight BMI and current dietary habits. Not surprisingly, physicians who have a higher level of awareness of their diet are always more likely to counsel them about nutrition and the importance of achieving a healthy weight. The physicians who have intentionally altered their diets are highly expected to help patients in making dietary changes.

BMI Calculation

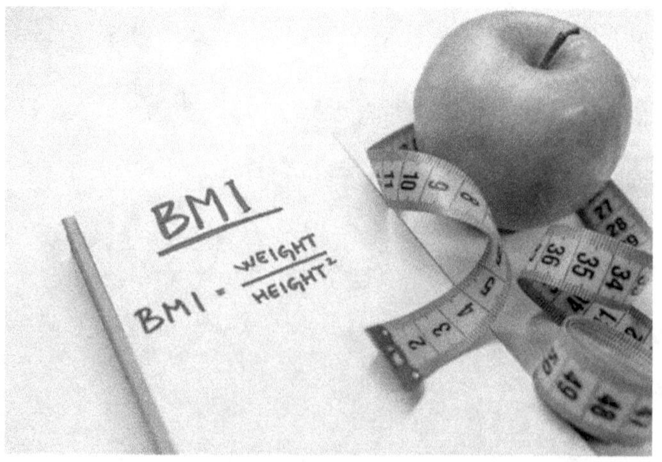

BMI is the contraction for body mass index. BMI Calculation is the calculated measurement based on height and weight, used as the screening tool for body fat, and identifies the potential health risks. BMI is not the exact measure of the body's composition, and it may be misleading, such as when used in professional's athletes. But it is a useful screening tool for a significant part of the population.

MyPlate 24 hours recall

For this part of your self-assessment, you must know:

- The types of all of the foods and beverages you had during the past day

- The method of food preparation

- The amount of each food item you have eaten

Interpret results and set goals

Using the tracker is just a great starting point to analyze the dietary intake but also remember:

- There are a few limitations of the food database.

- Difficulty in remembering or either estimating the portions eaten might affect the accuracy of the analysis.

If the past 24 hours aren't a typical day for your research might not reflect your overall diet quality.

Hence you can use your result as the general guidelines. For a more accurate analysis, you can try measuring and recording the intake at meals you have and also using the tracker for many days. After this, you only need to consider your results for the 24 hours recall and the recommendations and review the basic information presented at the beginning of this module. What have you learned through these recommendations of the analysis?

Set short and long-term achievable goals and also make a few healthy changes. Rather than creating a severe change in your diet, consider the modest changes that could provide you with more nutritious meals. Also, it would help if you considered the guidelines for any physical activity. Again, instead of only making severe changes that are not also sustainable, think about any typical day and its activities and then try to develop a workable plan that may increase the activity.

Little addictions in this activity may add up, such as parking a bit further at the end of the parking lot instead of only looking for the nearest spot you find in the area. Try to add a bit more time to the activities you enjoy doing the most, i.e., anything that gets you moving, such as walking, biking, and golf.

Dietary assessments are beneficial for the initial evaluation and are a great way for you to begin a conversation on diet and exercise habits. Patients with diet-regulated concerns or conditions must refer to the registered dietician for a thorough assessment and continuing care. So, are you ready to start building your life by being more food conscious and being healthy in life?

Conclusion

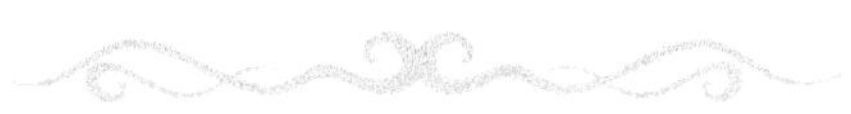

It can be difficult to maintain a healthier lifestyle, especially if you have grown up in an environment of junk food, crash diets, and no exercise. It can be both overwhelming and discouraging, so much so that you stop and return to your old ways in the middle of it, or you don't even bother in the first place. The common misconception in choosing such a lifestyle is that it's only done to lose weight or gain some abs. Yet, even better than that, you can do more than melt away your body fat by adopting a healthy lifestyle. A healthy lifestyle can improve your overall physical and mental health.

When you choose a safe lifestyle, you choose to be a happier person. Your physical health will be at its optimum level because you can shrink or gain into your ideal weight. Being slim is different from being healthy; it's not a good idea to be fat either. You are also vulnerable to multiple health complications, such as heart problems, hypertension, diabetes, stroke, and high blood pressure, whether you are too skinny or weigh twice as much as your ideal weight. But with a balanced diet - opting to eat nutritious meals and accompanied with moderate exercise - your physical health will be at its peak.

Also, you can improve your mental health by choosing a healthy lifestyle. Your brain cannot function well if you deprive yourself of food or do not consume the right amount of calories needed to fuel your body. But with a proper diet, you will be assured that you are getting all the necessary nutrients needed by your body. A good cardio exercise will also improve the circulation of blood in your system and improve your immune system, making you stronger and more focused each day. Just a brief 30-minute jog or run or an hour of yoga or Pilates will even help you focus and help fight depression and anxiety.

Choosing a healthy way of living is not an overnight process. It needs planning, hard work, and commitment to be able to achieve one. When you choose to change your lifestyle, you must be 100% committed to your plan, no matter how discouraging and tiring it can be. No change is simple and inviting at first, so you must set out your goals clearly and always focus on that trophy. You have to keep yourself motivated not to stop in the middle of your lifestyle change by going public and telling your family and friends about it or rewarding yourself now and then.

Thank You

www.ingramcontent.com/pod-product-compliance
Lightning Source LLC
Chambersburg PA
CBHW072300260726
48658CB00004BA/1303